To Thomas Glaser,

Best wishes in your career as group therapist and your ventures in Co-therapy.

Bill Roller & Vivian Nelson

# THE ART OF CO-THERAPY

# THE ART OF CO-THERAPY
## How Therapists Work Together

**Bill Roller, M.A.**
**Vivian Nelson, M.A.**
*Berkeley, California*

THE GUILFORD PRESS
London          New York

© 1991 The Guilford Press
A Division of Guilford Publications, Inc.
72 Spring Street, New York, NY 10012

Printed in the United States of America

This book is printed on acid-free paper

Last digit is print number: 9   8   7   6   5   4   3   2   1

**Library of Congress Cataloging-in-Publication Data**

Roller, Bill.
   The art of co-therapy: how therapists work together
/ Bill Roller, Vivian Nelson.
     p.  cm.
   Includes bibliographical references and index.
   ISBN 0-89862-557-2
   1. Multiple psychotherapy.   I. Nelson, Vivian.   II. Title.
RC489.M85R65     1991
616.89'14—dc20                   90-44744
                                        CIP

*Dedicated to*
*Virginia Satir*
*(1916–1988)*

◆　　◆

# Contents

Preface                                                                    xiii

Acknowledgments                                                              xv

**Introduction:**  A Relationship Book for Therapists          1
Definitions                                                                  2
Questions and Assumptions                                                    2
Dimensions of Our Inquiry                                                    4
Contents                                                                     5

## PART I: PRACTICING THE ART

**Chapter 1  Why Choose Co-Therapy?**                          11
The Meanings and Uses of Co-Therapy                                         11
   A definition of co-therapy   11
   Choosing a co-therapy relationship   12

Reasons for Selecting Co-Therapy                                           12
   Theoretical orientation of the therapists   12
   How patients bond with therapists   13

Benefits of the Co-Therapy Relationship                                    15
   Benefits that enhance therapist satisfaction and self-care   15
   Benefits that advance the treatment and enhance therapist
     satisfaction and self-care   17
   Benefits that advance the course of treatment   19
   Therapists and parents as models for human growth   21

Practical Considerations                                                   24
   Economy of effort and expense   24
   Practical aspects of complementarity   27

The Specific Nature of the Co-Therapy Relationship                         29
   The openly sexual co-therapy relationship   32
   The unequal team   35

**Chapter 2    Educational Reasons for Shared          37
                   Leadership**

Special Definitions for Unequal and Nontherapist          38
    Teams

Co-Therapy Research with Co-Learners, Nequipos,          40
    and Novice Co-Therapists

Rules for Supervisors                                     41
    Specific rules for therapists in nequipo teams   42
    Specific rules for supervisors of co-learners   42

The Learning Contract                                     43

Nequipo Teams in Action                                   46
    Acknowledging the assistant therapist   46
    An unacknowledged nequipo team   47
    A seductive assistant therapist   47
    Collusion with a patient's denial   48
    Training a family practice resident   50
    Co-therapists who became nequipos and vice-versa   51
    Training a member of the support staff   52

Co-Learner Teams in Action                                53
    A nequipo who became a co-learner   53
    Co-learners who hide their troubles from their supervisor   54
    Countertransference   55
    Competition with the supervisor   57
    Competition for the praise of the supervisor   58
    Supervisor's countertransference   59
    Co-dependency between co-learners   60

**Chapter 3    How to Choose a Co-Therapist              62**

Qualities that Therapists Desire in Co-therapists         63

Qualities that Therapists Bring to Co-Therapy             65

Sex as a Criterion for Choice                             68

Practical Instruments and Exercises for Selecting a       69
    Co-therapist

Co-Therapy Issues Questionnaire                           71

The Co-Therapy Contract                                   73

**Chapter 4    Why a Co-Therapy Team Becomes             75
                   Successful**

Complementary Balance of Skills                           76

Compatibility of Theoretical Viewpoints                   77

Openness in Communication                                 79

Equality of Participation                                 84

Liking Each Other                                         86

Respect 87

The Successful Co-Therapy Treatment of a Married
  Couple 88

The Successful Co-Therapy Treatment of a Family 91

**Chapter 5    Co-Therapy Teams in Trouble:** 96
**Impasses and Crises**

Definition of a Dysfunctional Team 97

Co-Therapists in Supervision 98

Co-Therapy Supervision with Ada and Jerry 99

The Five C's of Co-Therapy Dilemmas 100
  Competition   100
  Countertransference   106
  Confusion and lack of communication   112
  Lack of congruence between co-therapists   114
  Co-dependency between co-therapists   117

Special Problems and Vulnerability of Lovers and 121
  Marriage Partners Who Enter into Co-Therapy
  Relationships

Guidelines for Co-Therapy Couples 124

Secret Sexual Involvement of Co-Therapists 125

**Chapter 6    Treatment of a Borderline** 130
**and a Narcissistic Patient in**
**Co-Therapy**

Diagnostic Criteria 131

Treatment Options Unique to Co-Therapy 133

Psychodynamic Processes Worked Through by 133
  Co-Therapists

Christine 135
  The timing of reparenting in co-therapy treatment   138
  Co-therapist help with countertransference   140
  An example of projective identification   141
  More countertransference   142
  Loss of the special bond   143
  Why co-therapy now?   144

Kevin 145
  How co-therapists collaborate to manage their
    countertransference   145
  How co-therapy facilitated Kevin's changes in group   147
  Reparenting   149
  Concluding remarks on co-therapy treatment with
    Christine and Kevin   151

## PART II: MASTER PRACTITIONERS

**Chapter 7    Phases of Co-Therapy Team**          155
**Development**
*James M. Dugo and Ariadne P. Beck*

Introduction                                        155
Nine Phases of Co-Therapy Team Development          158
Phase 1: Creating a Contract                        163
    The seven issues as expressed in Phase 1    163
    Guidelines for institutions or group private practices
        regarding co-therapy    170
Phase 2: Forming an Identity                        172
    The seven issues as expressed in Phase 2    173
Phase 3: Building a Team                            179
    The seven issues as expressed in Phase 3    180
Conclusions                                         186

**Chapter 8    An Intimate Model for Co-Therapy**    189
*Robert L. Goulding and*
*Mary McClure Goulding*

Development as Person and Therapist                 190
    Establishment of a co-therapy team    193
Why Do Co-Therapy?                                  194
Disagreements                                       194
Comparable and Compatible                           195
Co-Therapy Is Not a Technique                       197
Experiences with Others as Co-Therapists            197
Male–Female Role Models                             198
Integration of Different Approaches                 199
Vignettes of Other Co-Therapy Teams                 200
Clients as "Co-Therapists"                          201
Training Therapists                                 201
Transference                                        203
Mistakes                                            204
Listening                                           204
Group Process                                       204
Hazards of Co-Therapy                               205
Advantages of Co-Therapy                            206
Who Benefits Most—Patients or Therapists?           208

**Chapter 9    Therapists and Parents as Models**    210
**for Being Human**
*Virginia Satir*

Every Child Is Asked to Choose                      213

Benefits                                                                      214

Difficulties                                                                  216

Co-Therapy Is a Means of Starting the Healing Process    218
   with Two People

Any Form of Therapy Can Work                                  219

**Appendix    Survey of the American Group            222
           Psychotherapy Association**
Co-therapy questionnaire   223
Results of the survey   224

Example of a Contract Between Nequipos                   232

Example of a Contract Between a Supervisor and       234
   Co-Learners

Table A. The Phases of Group Development               236

Table B. Emerging Leaders                                        237

**References**                                                            238

**Suggested Further Readings**                               243

**Index**                                                                    247

◆　◆

# *Preface*

With increasing numbers of psychotherapists entering the field over the past decade, there is a growing need for practical as well as theoretical information about psychotherapy. We have noted particularly the great interest shown in the topic of co-therapy during this time. Since most therapists will do co-therapy at some time during their career, particularly if they conduct family or group therapy (see Appendix, page 224), the need for guidance in this form of treatment has increased and will continue to do so.

This book is designed to provide basic information pertinent to the knowledge and skills required to practice co-therapy. Knowledge about how trained and experienced therapists practice co-therapy has been lacking to this point. Most research in the field has employed students and trainees as subjects. Consequently, the usefulness of findings has been limited. In this volume we publish for the first time the findings of our own national survey of co-therapy practices, attitudes, and beliefs among experienced psychotherapists in the field.

Remarkably, *The Art of Co-therapy: How Therapists Work Together* is the first book written on co-therapy. Many references to co-therapy have been made, but they exist in diverse places and in the texts of books not written specifically to address this topic. We believe that many therapists, whether currently practicing co-therapy or planning to do so in the future, have a need for a knowledgeable resource, a handbook to turn to in order to find information about co-therapy. The present volume attempts to satisfy that need.

We have placed the primary focus of our book on the co-therapy relationship, its creation, and the possibilities for therapeutic value that spring from its successful formation. Our goals are to describe how the co-therapy relationship can be established, to elaborate the criteria and prospects for its success, and to help practitioners problem solve in areas of identified difficulty.

Virginia Satir is the author of our final chapter, one of her last interviews before her death. Virginia was an early proponent of our project, and this volume is dedicated to her memory.

The vignettes we present herein are true stories derived from clinical practice but we have allowed ourselves fictional license in order to protect the identity of both client and therapist. To this end all names and situations have been altered significantly.

We hope that colleagues will find our text a challenging invitation to participate in a treatment practice that offers many rewards. We expect that practicing co-therapists will resonate to much of what we say and that we will stimulate discussion on a seminal topic neglected far too long.

*Berkeley, 1990*

BILL ROLLER
VIVIAN NELSON

# *Acknowledgments*

We wish to gratefully acknowledge the help of the following persons in the conceptualization, editing, and completion of this book: Virginia Satir for her initial support of our idea; Jim MacQueen for his astute criticism of Chapters 1 and 2; Fred Ilfeld and Barbara Squire for their excellent clinical examples; Jim Wolfe and Cynthia Scharlack for their careful reading of our text in the early stages; Jack Shonkwiler for his persistent encouragement over the years; Mark and Rebecca Apman for their assistance with the bibliography, and Mark especially for his input on nequipo and co-learner contracts; Jim Durkin for his timely information and suggestions; Steve Joseph, Michael Gray, and Pat McCaffrey for their thoughtful comments; and our fellow co-therapists and our trainees and, of course, our clients from whom we have learned so much.

Bill wants to give special recognition to Donald A. Shaskan, M.D., his co-editor of *Paul Schilder: Mind Explorer* (1985), and for many years his mentor in a nequipo team.

Bill and Vivian want to thank their siblings, Mary M. Roller and Jack P. Edelstein, who helped them learn the lessons of equality in their childhood.

$\blacklozenge$   $\blacklozenge$

# Introduction: A Relationship Book for Therapists

Whereas many books about making relationships have been written by therapists for their clients, this is the first book about making relationships written for therapists. The assumption that therapists know how to form working relationships with each other has seldom been challenged, and this explains in part why no book on co-therapy existed prior to the present volume. As therapists, we are trained to confront the underlying assumptions at work in the behavior of our patients; it is more difficult for us to see them at work in ourselves.

As a co-therapy team who became a married couple, we began our study with a lively and personal interest in the ability of psychotherapists to share the responsibility and authority of conducting psychotherapy. What made such a team work? How was co-therapy possible? These questions vivified our studies and motivated our workshops at the conferences of the Northern California Group Psychotherapy Society and the American Group Psychotherapy Association from 1978 to 1990. Our book has developed gradually over this period as an on-going dialogue among professionals who have helped fashion and shape its concepts. *The Art of Co-therapy: How Therapists Work Together* presents a particular point of view based on our experiences as co-therapists with each other and our co-therapy relationships and shared leadership experiences with 50 psychotherapists and trainees across 15 years of clinical practice. Our ideas have further been shaped by the 94 respondents to our nationwide random survey of American Group Psychotherapy Association members that we conducted in 1983 in order to assess current practices, attitudes, and beliefs held by experienced clinicians in the field.


## DEFINITIONS

The individual's relationship with his or her psychotherapist or the constellation of patients and their relationships with each other and their therapist define the mode of psychotherapy treatment. The four basic modes of psychotherapy treatment are individual therapy, family therapy, couple therapy, and group therapy. We define co-therapy as a special practice of psychotherapy in which two therapists treat a patient or patients in any mode of treatment at the same time and in the same place. Furthermore, co-therapy is a special practice of psychotherapy in which the relationship between the therapists is fundamental to the treatment process. Therapy involving multiple therapists of three or more is practiced, and therapy utilizing more than one therapist at different times for the same client, family, or group is also done. Both of these treatment conditions are beyond the scope of the present volume.


## QUESTIONS AND ASSUMPTIONS

Certain questions stand out in an inquiry such as ours. What does it mean to co-lead a task both for those following and for those leading? Why is such leadership desirable? What positive benefits are obtained? When might co-leadership become a burden to the leaders? When might it become harmful to those being led?

We begin by asking ourselves, "What are the chief characteristics of co-leadership and the sort of relationship it requires?" One assumption we make is prescriptive and has to do with equality. We suppose that co-leaders ought to share equally in their task. The equality we speak of may not consist in the kinds of jobs performed or even in the number of years of experience at the task. Rather it may consist in the time and energy expended and the degree of enthusiasm brought to the task. In Chapter 9, Virginia Satir states that equality is a matter of personal clarity.

> I believe you can be a garbage man and yet stand equal to others in value as a person if you are clear about what you know and what you do not know, what you can do and what you cannot do, and you value yourself. It is an issue of how congruent you are within yourself

and the degree of self-esteem you permit yourself. Clarity is the difference. Personal clarity allows equality to exist in the sense that a person is equal in value even though not equal in social status.

The "balancing" that so many of the respondents to our survey spoke of indicates a keen awareness of the principle of equality.

Another assumption we make is that co-therapy is not simply a technique that therapists employ. This assumption is radical and challenges many of the statements and definitions issued about co-therapy in the past (Lundin & Aronov, 1952; Rosenbaum, 1977, 1983). Co-therapy is a relationship in which two therapists embody and model, both verbally and non-verbally, emotional congruence, high self-esteem, and clear and direct communication.

Hannum (1980) has noted how rarely co-therapy has been defined as a form of treatment in and of itself, that is, a practice of psychotherapy that possesses its own unique set of techniques. We subscribe to this comprehensive view of co-therapy because it matches our perception of its depth and power. Some authors consider co-therapy "pivotal in the development of family therapy" (Napier & Whitaker, 1988, p. 56) and believe that "our co-therapy relationship is the basic instrument of therapy" (p. 91). Other authors (Rutan & Stone, 1984) give superficial treatment to the subject and seem to miss its profundity entirely. Such wide-ranging points of view are intriguing and remind us of the spectrum of human emotions that people bring to a work of art.

Co-therapy is a form of psychotherapy practice in which the relationship between the co-therapists becomes a crucial factor in both the healing process and the change process. It is not a technique. A technique implies an operation that can be applied and then discarded. Co-therapy is a commitment to a relationship with a peer in which significant therapeutic gains are possible for the patient and considerable collegial support and learning are possible for the therapists. If the co-therapy relationship is well made and the therapists have devoted time to its development, as they must, they will not so casually discard what they have created.

Many of the investigations reported in journal articles focus on the following question: with which clients and in what modes does co-therapy function best? Although these efforts are interesting and important, we believe that making hierarchical statements about where and when co-therapy should be employed as part of clinical practice, even if it could be done with a degree of certainty and exactitude, misses the critical point about what happens in the encounter between practitioners and clients. Co-therapy is a form of therapy in which the therapists themselves and their relationship with each other and their patients are the primary means of healing. This interactional matrix is responsible for the development, progress, and outcome of the therapy. This is the primary assumption and theoretical foundation on which our book rests.


## DIMENSIONS OF OUR INQUIRY

Throughout our study of co-therapy, we have been aware that we might be looking at a specific case of a more general phenomenon: co-leadership. Such a perspective has its limitations, yet it encourages the formation of general principles. Our work may be as much an essay on the functions of shared leadership as it is an essay on co-therapy. How do we define leadership?

> Leadership over human beings is exercised when persons with certain motives and purposes mobilize, in competition or conflict with others, institutional, political, psychological, and other resources so as to arouse, engage, and satisfy the motives of followers. This is done in order to realize goals mutually held by both leaders and followers. . . . Leaders do not obliterate followers' motives though they may arouse certain motives and ignore others . . . To control things. . . . is an act of power, not leadership, for things have no motives. Power wielders may treat people as things. Leaders may not. (Burns, 1978, p. 18)

Burns' emphasis on motives is germane to our study. Leaders must embody the motives of those who follow them lest they forfeit their relevance and persuasiveness. Yet, leaders must also remain true to their own vision and put forward their own motives and purposes in the form of action. The presence of conflict is also pertinent, since leaders must always compete with alternative and sometimes opposite directives and messages from parents, society, peers, and other sources of influence. Co-leaders must comprehend the motives and conflicts of those who follow them.

It is both desirable and advisable to share many tasks in ordinary life. Parenting is one such task. When we exclude the clinical material that deals with pathology and patient care, most of the ideas we formulate regarding the relationship between co-therapists can readily be applied to the relationship between parents who desire to co-parent their children in equal fashion.

Some people in business are now experimenting with co-leadership in order to discover the beneficial and profitable results of mutual collaboration (Barnett & Barnett, 1988). Frank and Deborah Popper have recently demonstrated the efficacy of a co-equal research team in land use planning (Matthews, 1990). Do these nonclinical situations have things in common with the focus of our study? We believe our findings may help to explain why co-leadership—real co-leadership—is so rare in the world of work in general. We believe we are part of a new trend of professionals who want to explore the secrets of partnership success and truly wish to share leadership in the workplace.

## CONTENTS

Part I is an overview of the subject of co-therapy. We have taken our survey as a starting point to examine the various aspects of co-therapy. Yet, we have used the data creatively to stimulate our own thinking on the subject. We trust that the dialectic between these two tendencies, the desire to remain true to our subjects' reports and the desire to extend and develop new theory in the field, provides a fruitful and practical synthesis for our readers.

The opening chapter defines co-therapy and gives reasons why a therapist would choose to practice it. Chapter 2 introduces special definitions for unequal and nontherapist teams that have been organized for teaching purposes and gives guidelines to training programs and supervisors who employ these methods. Chapter 3 examines the many aspects of choosing a co-therapist. We provide questionnaires and other tools to assist in that process. Chapter 4 delineates the positive signs for success of a co-therapy team and describes the successful treatment of a married couple and a family. In Chapter 5, we discuss co-therapy teams in trouble and describe a number of teams at impasses and in crises. We offer practical ways to anticipate dilemmas and solve problems. In Chapter 6, we present co-therapy in action as we trace our treatment of a borderline personality and a narcissistic personality.

In Part II, other co-therapy teams take a different tack to both augment and elucidate the major premises of the book. James Dugo and Ariadne Beck propose a fascinating model for viewing the co-therapy relationship as a developing system. The co-therapy relationship develops incrementally over time and will do so under the influence of a particular treatment group and its specific institutional or private practice setting. Then, Robert and Mary Goulding take a highly personal approach to their experiences with co-therapy over twenty years of practicing together as a husband–wife team. Their subjective impressions and clinical observations illuminate and expand on many of the comments offered by the psychotherapists in our survey. Finally, Virginia Satir raises her inimitable voice to make some exquisite and provocative statements about co-therapy and the nature of the therapy process itself.

In closing, we want to emphasize four points. First, we believe it is essential for a person to have the experience of doing therapy alone with individuals, groups, couples, and families. The learning and impact of such exposure is undeniably central to the training of a therapist. Co-therapy does not substitute for it.

Second, we want to point out that co-therapy is not a new practice. In the 1920s, Alfred Adler (1930) first experimented with employing two counselors instead of one to break through resistances in the treatment of children in the presence of their parents at his Child Guidance Clinic in Vienna. The child sometimes responded better when two persons, a psychiatrist and either a social worker or teacher, discussed the child's circumstances in his or her presence.* The first psychotherapy group with adults in a hospital setting in the United States was co-led. That group was conducted at Bellevue Hospital in 1936 with Paul Schilder and Donald Shaskan (Shaskan & Roller, 1985; Roller, 1986) sharing the leadership.

Third, some of what we have to say about co-therapy is an elaboration of what others have said before, but in less precise and less organized form. The literature reveals much in the way of opinion and little in the way of well-researched facts. Calls have been issued for a definitive study of co-therapy, its effectiveness and its dynamics. These calls have largely been unanswered. The present study, although far from being definitive, is one response to a need so often expressed.

Fourth, we believe that those persons who want to understand the deeper, internal processes that go on within the mind of the solo therapist can learn much by observing the interactions and dialogue between co-therapists. The transactions of a co-therapy team replicate the dialectical reasoning and inner conflict that goes on inside the mind of the clinician. In this manner, the internal work of the therapist is made transparent and the reader may gain unexpected insights into the workings of the therapist's mind by the study of co-therapists' inter-actions. By our analysis of co-therapists' interactions in Chapters 4 and 5 we provide examples of this phenomenon, and in Chapter 6 we offer more opportunities to look at the same phenomenon in the treatment of patients with disturbed object relations.

We do have a definite bias in favor of co-therapy as a method of treatment and advocate its use. We do not, however, claim that co-therapy is better than solo treatment in any modality; nor do we claim that co-therapy is the treatment of choice for any particular kind of

*Alexandra Adler, personal correspondence, September 28, 1987.

client. Yet, even in the absence of clear outcome research that indicates the effectiveness of the co-therapy variable in the treatment of patients, the number of therapists practicing co-therapy increases with each passing year. We have written this book to respond to the very practical needs of those therapists embarking on the task of co-leadership and those faced with the immediate challenge of working out a co-therapy relationship.

Future researchers may find empirical evidence to suggest that many of our assumptions about co-therapy are wrong. For example, we assume that co-therapy, under certain conditions we prescribe, can be therapeutic or at least can facilitate the progress of the therapy of our clients. Yet, it may be found that therapists themselves gain most from the practice and that other conditions such as positive reinforcement, astute interventions, and timely interpretations may prove to be more pertinent to healing. We also assume that as co-therapy teams learn to function better and co-therapists mature in their relationships with each other, so they can be more available therapeutically in the treatment of their patients. Although this statement seems intuitively valid, it may not prove true and may only beg the question that co-therapy itself is effective treatment.

However, until that time when the experts at last arrive to dispel our ignorance, we as clinicians must face the daily responsibility of caring for our clients. We believe it is both ethically and clinically sound to prepare ourselves as co-therapists to provide treatment for our patients in the absence of sure knowledge of our effectiveness and to avoid as rigorously as possible doing them harm. We wager that pragmatic considerations alone make our project a worthwhile effort. With this modest aim in mind and the desire to improve the practical knowledge available to co-therapists and would-be co-therapists, we submit the following ideas and hope they will prove helpful.

# ◆ PART I ◆

# Practicing the Art

# ◆ 1 ◆

# *Why Choose Co-Therapy?*

## THE MEANINGS AND USES OF CO-THERAPY

### *A Definition of Co-Therapy*

Co-therapy is a special practice of psychotherapy in which two or more therapists treat one or more patients in group, family, couple, or individual psychotherapy at the same time and in the same place.* It is a form of psychotherapy treatment in which the therapist relates not only to a patient or patients but also to a peer or peers. Co-therapy is essentially a professional relationship that has the potential to develop and deepen over time and to affect and alter profoundly the lives of its practitioners. When we use co-therapy in this book, we mean just *two* therapists at work. The prospect of more than two therapists working simultaneously together is fascinating but complicated and beyond the scope of the present volume. In 1983, we conducted a co-therapy survey of the American Group Psychotherapy Association (see Appendix). Although we defined co-therapy as "two or more therapists working conjointly" in the questionnaire for our survey, it was clear from their responses that our sample was speaking almost exclusively of dyadic co-therapy teams. We assumed that co-therapy was most commonly practiced among group therapists, and we wanted to learn the standard of practice and beliefs of experienced clinicians in the field.

---

*One exception to our definition is the case in which individuals contract to work together for the sake of learning how to practice psychotherapy. Learning contracts established between non-peers and peers who are not therapists are discussed in detail in Chapter 2.

We were pleased to discover that not only was our random sample highly experienced as clinicians, but three quarters of them possessed in-depth experience as co-therapists.

### Choosing a Co-Therapy Relationship

Therapists choose co-therapy primarily because the co-therapy relationship benefits both the clincians and patients. We want to emphasize that, in choosing co-therapy, one not only selects a special practice of psychotherapy but also chooses a relationship. We believe the choice of a relationship has direct consequences for the treatment of patients. We also believe the specific nature of the relationship affects patient care. Situations in which a supervisor and a trainee or two trainees together constitute the co-therapy dyad are special cases that do not meet our criteria for co-therapy. They are frequently applied as teaching methods for therapists in training and will be discussed separately in Chapter 2, "Educational Reasons for Shared Leadership."

The relationships that develop in co-therapy grow out of the particular circumstances and preferences of each co-therapy team and reflect two dimensions: (1) the theoretical orientation of the therapists and (2) the notion of how patients bond with their therapists.

## REASONS FOR SELECTING CO-THERAPY

### Theoretical Orientation of the Therapists

The increased opportunity for learning that comes from discussion and collaboration with a peer was the reason for co-therapy selection most frequently stated in our survey. Two persons may agree to work together because they share a similar theoretical framework and hope to build a partnership on this common basis. Therapists may also seek others who differ from themselves in knowledge and orientation in the hope of learning new skills and adding to their own depth. The question becomes, "How similar or different must the peer be for me to gain from collaboration?" Too much similarity poses no challenge, whereas too much difference feeds frustration and pointless conflict.

Looking at the comments by the respondents to our survey, it is clear that co-therapists learn a lot from each other. Sharing and learning are reciprocated to a large degree because therapists expressly state that these are two reasons why they sought a co- therapy relationship in the first place. The learning may be "cognitive," but experiential learning seems to be valued more. Many therapists refer to co-therapy as a "good learning model," particularly where each therapist has more depth and breadth of experience in different areas than his or her partner. "It keeps the therapy more interesting" was a typical comment. "Co-therapy provides on-going discussion and peer supervision that mutually enhance therapy skills." The opportunity to share feedback and collaborate is greatly desired.

The second reason most often cited for choosing co-therapy as the form of treatment was the widened perspectives afforded a therapist by having a peer observing the same events of the therapy. Having another look at the same phenomenon can open the door to different intervention options. This can be most desirable when a therapist is at an impasse with a client. It is generally desirable as a way to increase pathways to change for the health of the client. Again, the therapist must decide how tolerant he or she can be with widely differing points of view. A new perspective can be welcome, but only if the therapist can be open to hearing and seeing its value. A critical balance must be struck between perspectives that challenge a therapist's formulations and perspectives that are irreconcilable with those formulations. The latter may prove more confusing than helpful for the patient.

Each opportunity for greater learning and widened perspective carries with it at least the possibility for dispute if the new input falls too far from the center of one's own beliefs. There are real limitations to our flexibility as people and co-therapists, and this must be considered in the choices we make.

A co-therapist can also correct for emotional and perceptual bias in the other. Thus, two views of personality problems and dynamics can be obtained instead of one and the co-therapy relationship offers the opportunity for a wider point of view. But this presumes that each is willing and able to assert his or her own point of view. And that presumes co-therapists who possess high self-esteem and confidence in their diagnostic and clinical skills. They must trust that their partner will respect another opinion. They must be able to listen closely to a different point of view and give serious thought to how a patient, a family, or a group might be described and treated differently.

### How Patients Bond with Therapists

How patients will relate to their therapists and what the nature of that bond will be is a crucial factor in the choice of co-therapy. The respondents in our survey listed widened transference possibilities for patients as their third most important reason for selecting the practice of co-therapy. But this reason makes sense only if one accepts the idea that transference is a desired relationship between client and therapist at some point in the therapy. If the idea of patient bonding or nonbonding with therapists is not shared to some degree by co-therapists, the goals they hope to obtain by practicing co-therapy can be severely compromised. In this case, they may find themselves on the road to co-therapy dysfunction and put their patients at risk. Pertinent questions for co-therapists are:

1. How available emotionally will you make yourself to your clients?
2. How willing are you to let transference flower?
3. How much will you relate to your client as a person and how much as an authority figure?
4. Operationally, what is your preferred psychological distance with clients?

If co-therapists hope to establish by their collaboration more targets for patients to project onto, they are clearly indicating the desirability of transference as part of the curative process. For example, a male–female co-therapy team can become powerful mother–father objects for their families, individual clients, or members of their groups. One outcome of such a therapeutic strategy might be safety and protection for those clients who had been abused by their own parents in their families of origin. Another outcome of such a strategy might be the opportunity for a patient to gain acceptance and love from her therapist-father without the fear of losing the therapist-mother's approval and love. In both cases, the opportunity for clients to work through these early childhood conflicts in therapy can be intensified greatly by dual transference objects.

The presence of an additional transference target can activate early memories of family scenes. Even with same-sex co-therapists, clients often choose one therapist to be their mother and the other their father, or brother, or sister, without respect to the sex of the therapists.

In particular, a male and female combination creates a family structure that can prove quite useful. Elizabeth Mintz (1963, pp. 127–132) has noted that ". . . special difficulties in relating to either male or female authority figures can be worked through by patients who would have been unwilling to choose a therapist of the more threatening sex."

However, if the co-therapists do not intend to foster transference as a goal of co-therapy, there is still the question of what kind of bond they will form. How much will they allow their patients to see them as people and how much as experts in the field? Even if the roles as parents are eschewed, what distinct and valuable lessons can therapists provide in the co-therapy form of treatment?

## BENEFITS OF THE CO-THERAPY RELATIONSHIP

The benefits reported by therapists in our survey are summarized in the following categories:

1. A greater opportunity for learning through discussion and collaboration with a therapist.
2. Widened perspectives for therapists.
3. Widened transference possibilities for patients.
4. Greater learning opportunities for patients.
5. Opportunity for therapists to check and balance their complementary behavior.

The first two benefits are specific to therapists and enhance therapist satisfaction and self-care. The next two are specific to patients and advance the course of treatment. The last seems to favor both therapists and patients. These five concepts appeared with greater frequency than any other benefits mentioned by our respondents. We shall expand on these and other benefits and also include pertinent remarks by other investigators.

We propose two ways of viewing the possible benefits of the co-therapy relationship: co-therapy indicated for reasons of therapist satisfaction and self-care and co-therapy indicated for clinical reasons to advance the course of treatment. These two overlap to some extent. Clinically skillful and appropriate interventions that help patients can be most satisfying for therapists. And it can be assumed that a satisfied and nurtured therapist can be more clinically available to his or her patients.

### Benefits that Enhance Therapist Satisfaction and Self-Care

We have already addressed some ways co-therapy benefits the practitioner. There are a few additional benefits we can add. It is easier for co-therapists to sustain the loss of a family after sudden and premature termination of family therapy. If the therapists have devoted much energy to the treatment of the family, the effect can be emotionally gut wrenching to believe that their efforts were unproductive and perhaps even harmful. The co-therapists can console one another and share in the mourning process of their hopes for the family. This process helps them gain a balance of perspective since their hopes for treatment may have been greatly exaggerated and unrealistic in retrospect. The primary bond of the co-therapists is with each other, not with the family, and so their loss is ameliorated. In this respect and others, the therapists can gratify each other so they will not seek gratification from their patients (Whitaker, Warkentin, & Johnson, 1950).

Therapists need acknowledgment and appreciation for work well done. A mature co-therapy team is able to provide mutual acknowledgment for accomplishment. This ability adds greatly to the job satisfaction of the therapists and reinforces their interest and willingness to continue the co-therapy relationship and reinforces their interest in co-therapy in general. This benefit served as a chief motivator for therapists to conduct group psychotherapy at the Group Health Cooperative of Puget Sound, a large health maintenance organization in Washington state (Roller, Schnell, & Welsch, 1982) where it proved to be of great value in the development of the group psychotherapy program. Co-therapy teams deepen their relationships over time and learn new ways to balance their strengths and weaknesses as co-leaders. When this occurs, a tremendous incentive for continuing group psychotherapy is set in motion. Co-therapists like to be together so they start more groups—and the more groups they begin, the more they learn to like each other.

Co-therapy also provides an edge in the prevention of burnout among a staff. In a mental health delivery system, therapists tend to become so intently focused on the demands of their own practice that they may become increasingly isolated from the parallel work of their colleagues. Co-leadership allows therapists the opportunity to work side by side with their colleagues and exchange ideas as well as emotional support. A countertransference reaction, so prevalent as a factor in the burnout syndrome, can be discussed and worked through with the aid of a co-therapist, either in or outside of the treatment session.

Co-therapy provides companionship for practitioners and a bulwark against professional loneliness. The practice of psychotherapy, especially in a private setting, is a lonely and isolating experience for many. Although therapists work with people, the stance of the therapist is listening and giving attention. Reciprocity in these activities is neither expected nor appropriate from a client. Since co-therapists are peers, they are able to do these things for each other.

Co-therapy is a source of emotional support for practitioners. For example, a therapist who is questioning his or her own approach or strategy with a difficult patient or a family can find encouragement from a co-therapist. A member of an experienced co-therapy team knows how his or her partner works, and this knowledge facilitates brief and informal consultation. This is especially important in the face of extraordinary therapeutic demands. When faced with powerful psychopathology, co-therapists can "better withstand the assault of delusional systems" (Russell & Russell, 1979, pp. 39–46). They can "reality test" with each other to prevent their enmeshment in the psychotic process. Also, they can keep each other from yielding to the belief that there is no solution, a belief so characteristic of dysfunctional families.

Co-therapists grow personally by their collaboration. One positive outcome of their personal growth is their increased enthusiasm for psychotherapy.

### Benefits that Advance the Treatment and Enhance Therapist Satisfaction and Self-Care

One focus of the debate surrounding co-therapy traditionally has been the question "Who benefits more, patient or therapist?" We make no attempt to answer this question for two reasons. First, although this is an important and natural question to ask, it does not convey a full understanding of what therapy is about. Therapy is not a lottery situation where, if the therapist wins, the patient loses. The relationship is more complex than that. Second, the question appears impossible to answer and only begs the question that co-therapy itself is beneficial. We recognize that some elements of co-therapy do address the patients' interests more directly and others address those of the practitioners. We have organized our thinking along these lines as we have written this chapter. But we also understand that our choices on this matter are subjective, and other judgments may be equally valid. The following elements appear to us to benefit both sides of the therapeutic encounter.

Co-therapists can help each other stay centered and avoid problematic countertransference issues. They may be able to see in each other some of their own unresolved problems that linger and affect their ability to function as therapists. Their facility in pointing to these problem areas will depend on their degree of trust and respect for each other, the maturity of the co-therapy team, and how far they have advanced as partners (see Chapter 7). The capacity to see difficulties is a function of astute observation and personal awareness; the capacity to discuss difficulties with each other is a function of the partners' development as a co-therapy team and their ability to communicate.

Another important advantage is that there is less likelihood that two therapists will be manipulated by the family in therapy. As Luthman and Kirschenbaum (1974) note:

> With two therapists in operation, it is almost impossible for a family to manipulate the therapy situation for any appreciable length of time, if at all. Usually, when one is working, the other is observing

and can be particularly attuned to the nonverbal behavior in the family. Or, the other can take space to tune into his subjective experience of being with the family and pick up on fantasy or imagery clues. (p. 193)

"Two observers contribute to greater objectivity," is a common belief expressed by the co-therapists in our survey. Co-therapists can arrive at a consensus about what is really occurring in the therapy. One therapist's negative judgments about a particular person in a family or group can be balanced by the perceptions of his or her partner. One therapist may indulge or ignore a patient's acting out, but his or her co-therapist can raise the issue into the consciousness of the patient. Together, the team can avoid being sucked into the system and thereby lessen the chance of enmeshment with the family or group. David Rubenstein and Oscar Weiner (1967) corroborate our respondents' remarks. "A single therapist can be seduced into sharing and confirming the most bizarre of family beliefs. The presence of a co-therapist helps to prevent this possibility." Therapists can talk to each other and overcome a sense of helplessness that may permeate family therapy sessions.

By skillful collaboration, co-therapists also can gauge a family's resistance to change and monitor the family's attempts to enmesh the therapists. Minuchin, Montalvo, Guerney, Rossman, and Schumer (1967, p. 288) state:

Whenever one therapist is involved in interaction with a family, the cotherapist's field of observation includes the therapist, not just the family alone. He learns to watch specifically for the ways in which the family organizes his partner into behaving along lines which do not permit family change.

Co-therapists are able to take greater risks in the use of themselves as a means of healing without fear of being swallowed by their powerful countertransference responses. Minuchin and Fishman (1981, pp. 30–31) discuss how Whitaker manages this process.

Carl Whitaker's solution to the problem of maintaining therapeutic leverage is to have a co-therapist: "I don't think one therapist alone possesses the amount of power necessary to get in and change the family and get back out again. . . . I don't want to stay the rest of my life with my finger stuck in the dike." With a co-therapist, the therapist can then solve his "countertransference problem by re-treating into his relationship to the other therapist, and the thera-peutic process then becomes a process of the two groups relating to each other." Whitaker trusts the "we," his co-therapist and himself, while not always trusting either of them alone; together they have "stereoscopic vision." With the protection of the co-therapist, Whitaker, whose goal is a creative expansion for the family and for himself, enters into an intense personal involvement with the family, accepting the family impact on the therapist as inevitable and frequently beneficial.

## Benefits that Advance the Course of Treatment

Patients can learn about relationships as they watch two persons, both equal in power and self-esteem, model how to behave as individuals in a relationship. Our survey respondents clearly noted this phenomenon, and they cited greater learning opportunities for their patients as a boon of co-therapy. Since patients can identify with either or both therapists, co-therapy can enhance the patients' ability to explore and reveal the many psychological parts of themselves. How does that happen? Patients can discover and reveal multiple facets of their personalities as they relate differently to each co-therapist. For example, a woman may want to practice her assertiveness by challenging the male therapist and deepen her self-acceptance as a woman by receiving nurturing from the female therapist. Both can occur.

Co-therapists can model different kinds of behavior for a client to follow. A client can see the co-therapists' different responses to a single stimulus and learn that probably there is more than one choice that is right. A client can see that there are many pathways to the same goal, and his or her judgment and decision making can thereby improve. For example, the client can experiment with the style of communication of one therapist and then try that of the other therapist to see which fits better. Clients can experience a greater depth in their own personalities, since they are presented with two mirrors, two reflections of themselves to contemplate. In this way, they achieve a better integration of their personalities.

When a patient has been in individual treatment with one of the therapists of a co-therapy team, the introduction of that patient to treatment by co-therapy in a group setting usually reveals new information about the patient's dynamics. There are two factors that change: the addition of a second therapist and the patient's admission into a group of peers. We see the first factor most clearly when together we conduct interviews with the patient prior to his or her entry into our group. The interview usually has diagnostic value. For example, we have seen a patient experience a greater awareness of her dependency on Vivian, her individual therapist, and a heightened fear of her dependence as it became more obvious in the presence of Bill. We predicted that the patient might become counterdependent in group psychotherapy to demonstrate her autonomy. We discussed how best to proceed given this insight into her emotional response to dependency. We have also seen a client become quite regressed and frightened during a first interview in co-therapy. This is often a sign that the client is not ready to enter co-therapy treatment in group. He or she may require co-therapy sessions as an individual first in order to work through his or her fear. He or she may fear a member of the opposite sex or, specifically, an authority figure of the opposite sex. These aspects of the client's personality might have remained undisclosed, if the patient had not entered treatment in co-therapy. Dreikurs, Shulman, and Mosak (1952a) described this phenomenon quite succinctly:

> Individual psychotherapy takes place in an artificial atmosphere which may permit the patient to adjust to the limited relationship with one person, often through an emotional involvement. The introduction of a third person often upsets this equilibrium and may result in the patient's revealing more of his natural reactions. This permits both therapists to evaluate the patient's attitudes and progress. Patients sometimes remain on very good behavior through a desire to please the active therapist. The presence of the second therapist is often disturbing enough to the structure of the situation so that the patient is more likely to exhibit more fully his disturbed relationships with people. (p. 221)

Clients can see how two very different—or very similar—persons forge a relationship over time. They can see two persons interrelate in a mature relationship that is open, creative, and in which both are able to enjoy the comfort of familiarity.

Co-therapy softens the tyranny of one. It helps differentiate the therapists into distinct persons, neither omniscient nor omnipotent. It helps destroy the illusion that the therapist is an all-knowing magus. We elaborate further on this subject in our discussion of the narcissistic therapist in Chapter 5, page 121.

A co-therapist can correct misperceptions by his or her partner and counterbalance his or her excesses. For example, the indulgent therapist can rely on his or her critical partner to give frank assessments of their patients' capabilities, a valuable step in developing a treatment plan and prognosis. The critical therapist can rely on the indulgent partner to support and nurture the self-esteem of poorly achieving clients, an important step in helping them experience self-acceptance.

Role flexibility is another desirable characteristic. For example, one therapist can be active and the other can monitor, and then, later, alternate roles. One can sit back and think while the other is intensely involved. One can be playful while the other is serious. Co-therapists can mollify each other's rigid habits in group by challenging each other's customary roles. For example, a therapist might be very sedate and passive in a group of homogeneously depressed patients until the arrival of a co-therapist who pushes for more activity, movement, and playfulness. This may prove to be a productive change in the service of the patients' treatment. "My co-therapist keeps me on alert and critically thinking about my work," is a typical comment.

Along with role flexibility there is opportunity to be flexible in therapeutic approach at a particular time. In group therapy, one therapist can do individual therapy with a group member, while the co-therapist watches the group process and comments on how the individual work affects the group. This is also true in couple therapy, where one therapist addresses one client while the other therapist looks for affect in the other client.

Co-therapists can be more available to patients at crucial times in treatment. When a family member individuates dynamically from marital symbiosis as a result of family therapy, the behavior of the individuating member can change suddenly.

> But it is important to realize that the family system is thrown out of balance by the individuation and that other family members need help, too. The mounting anxiety in the "immobile" spouse is an especially critical element. As these sometimes dramatic shifts are attempted late in the therapy process, the therapists must be available to everyone in the family and to all the relationships. At such a time we are more aware than ever of the need for co-therapy. (Napier & Whitaker, 1988, p. 234)

Co-therapy permits synergy to flourish. Synergy was conceptualized by our respondents as a synthesis of the skills and knowledge of two persons. The formula for synergy is expressed as $1 + 1 > 2$. In this formula the combination augments and expands the capabilities of both. Dugo and Beck believe this begins to occur in Phase 3 of co-therapy development (see Chapter 7). A mature co-therapy team brings energy into a group and brings new life to the leadership function.

### Therapists and Parents as Models for Human Growth

Modeling allows co-therapists to magnify the impact of the therapeutic encounter in a way not possible by solo practice. They are able to model transactional and interpersonal behavior between peers for their clients. We speak of modeling not in the simple sense of imitation but in the larger sense of the transfer of qualities to clients. By this means, a special kind of learning takes place. In Chapter 4 we describe the treatment of a couple to whom we transferred our qualities of toleration and respect. Indeed, the effect of modeling in shaping human behavior and attitudes is often profound. Poets have recognized the close relationship between a model to fashion oneself by and the creative spirit within the individual (Snyder, 1983):

> In making the handle
> Of an axe
> By cutting wood with an axe
> The model is indeed near at hand.*
>
> (LU JI, *Wen Fu*, 4th century C.E.)

A co-therapy team coaches and teaches by example the exquisite crafting of human relationships. The one-to-one therapy situation, where a single therapist treats an individual patient, demonstrates some of the same healing effects for patients that are possible with co-therapy. However, the relationship formed is not between equals. Co-therapy strives foremost to be a relationship between equals. To that purpose, co-therapists accept the challenge to create something that is special and difficult and a gift to their patients.

Whitaker makes the parallel between parenting and co-therapy in the following way: "I think of it (co-therapy) as the father and mother pattern. . . . It is the team that is the therapist, not the individual. I don't believe there is such a thing as a 'single parent'; it takes two people to parent children. And with the team pattern, the essential characteristic is the necessity for mutual respect . . ." (Whitaker & Garfield, 1987, p. 110).

Both co-therapy and parenting begin with the image and symbol of two in relationship. A relationship of two can bring about a third unique creation. This is a principle of biology and sexual propagation. The desire to pair and communicate is a principle of psychology. In parenting and co-therapy, the symbol is two in relationship with a third at a distance watching and learning. Openness between two can create a space for a third person, and that third person can become whole and unique and valuable in him- or herself.

Parents provide the human being with his or her first opportunity to see an equal, sharing, and supportive dyad. Parents can share the tasks of child watching and rearing. Although their functions may be different, their responsibility for the child's well-being can be shared equally

*Excerpted from *Axe Handles*, copyright 1983 by Gary Snyder. Published by Northpoint Press and reprinted by permission.

if the parents trust, respect, and empower each other. They can practice congruence with each other, which is to say they can state what they know and what they don't know. They can ask directly, "I don't know how to do this with our child . . . Can you help?" Or, one can offer, "I know a little about fishing for a child's imagination . . . Let me try to reach her with this story." Such generous attitudes produce benefits for their child because several pathways to a desired goal may be laid out by both parents, and the child can choose among them. Since each parent can have equal self-worth, the child is not forced to choose one parent over the other simply to be loyal or boost the parent's self-esteem.

In like fashion, truly equal co-therapists offer twice as many options to their client. The client is free to choose what fits him or her best, knowing that the self-esteem of his or her therapists does not depend on how he or she has chosen. Co-therapists model communication between equals. Either therapist can say directly to his or her partner, "I was wrong about that. Do you have a better idea?" For example, the client can benefit from hearing a male therapist discuss his view about being a son. The client can watch as the therapist turns to his female counterpart and asks, "What do you find to be true among daughters?" The client can watch the male listening and learning from his female partner.

The value and utility of open disagreement can be demonstrated as well. If both are equal, then both can have equal standing in a disagreement about theory or approach or technique. The fundamental agreement here is that disagreement will be openly acknowledged and will not threaten the personal value of either party, nor will it diminish the amount of attention the client receives.

Modeling by therapists consists largely of nonverbal actions, which are seldom missed by those in treatment. Patients in treatment with solo therapists are acutely aware of the nuances in their therapists' character and behavior. In co-therapy treatment, patients are careful watchers and listeners who take in every subtlety and nuance of the co-therapists' relationship. For example, body image and posture are ways of picturing one's body and carrying oneself (Schilder, 1985). The body images and posture evinced by two persons who are both equal in self-worth and congruent in their acceptance of their own abilities and limitations are striking to observe. We immediately see teamwork in action and recognize the hallmarks of competence: economy of energy in the service of intelligent strategy. Things get done. Children receive needed attention and yet are not overindulged by parents seeking to prove their own self-worth. Clients learn that grandiosity and depression are products of an unaccepting self.

Although our model for co-therapy is a man and a woman in a relationship, other possibilities exist. Same-sex co-therapy teams are numerous, and we give examples of their work as we describe the lives of co-therapy teams. Although we write exclusively about hetero-sexual co-therapists, we believe the elements for successful co-therapy apply to homosexual co-therapists as well. Many of the issues that heterosexual teams face are identical to those encountered by homo-sexual teams. We believe there are certain aspects of the male–female dyad that recommend it for specific kinds of treatment, such as repa-renting, and we elaborate on these when we describe our reparenting of Christine in Chapter 6.

## PRACTICAL CONSIDERATIONS

Therapists choose co-therapy secondarily because of practical consid-erations such as convenience and shared resources. There is some overlap with clinical reasons for doing co-therapy at this level as well, since many sound clinical procedures have utility and practicality as their raisons d'être.

After studying the results of our survey, we came to a striking conclusion: more than just hazards prevent therapists from choosing co-therapy, and more than just benefits inspire clinicians to its practice. There are other conditions that influence psychotherapists' decisions in this regard. Some of these conditions are captured in the following questions: How much effort am I willing to spend in order to find a suitable person and establish a working contract? Can I afford the time and effort it takes? Can I lessen some of the demands on my time by sharing patient responsibility with a co-therapist? How suitable am I for co-therapy? What if I truly prefer to do group or family therapy alone? What if I find co-therapy too complicated for the context of my practice? Can my clients afford the additional cost?

In our survey we gathered nearly twice as many beneficial com-ments about co-therapy than statements pointing to hazards. This betrayed a strong sample bias toward co-therapy. It also pointed to a flaw in our survey. We asked for an enumeration of hazards but did not ask "What prevents you from doing co-therapy?" It is important to remember that there are reasons for choosing co-therapy that have little to do with clinical indications or therapist satisfaction. We de-scribe some of these practical issues below.

### Economy of Effort and Expense

In our survey, therapists expressed a belief that both their patients and themselves experienced greater logistic support when a co-therapy team was in operation. Two therapists are more available than one to take telephone calls and schedule extra individual appointments. Therapists are able to share the work and responsibility of forming and sustaining a group. The energy necessary to sustain group psychotherapy practice over time is considerable, and co-therapists can share both the effort and costs of marketing their group. The effort to start a group is especially demanding. Co-therapists can feed referrals into one group from two practices.

Having a backup therapist reduces anxiety for the co-therapist. The idea of having coverage for an individual, group, or family by a professional who has both shared experience with and knowledge of the patients is most attractive. The continuity of care for the group or family is guaranteed when one therapist is ill or on vacation. A co-therapist can stop performing maintenance tasks temporarily for a group in full knowledge that the group will continue because his or her peer will pick up the slack. He or she will not lose income because of absence; thus, co-therapists in private practice provide a measure of economic security for each other. The idea that quality work can be accomplished when it is shared can be quite liberating. It is a statement of both maturity and humility to acknowledge that one therapist cannot be all things to his or her patients.

Co-therapists can share the difficult interventions and confrontations necessary in good psychotherapy and shoulder the consequences of inevitable mistakes. One example is the need to confront the patient who was sexually abused as a child and is now at risk of becoming an offender. To miss this diagnosis entirely and perhaps not even ask questions relevant to abuse are unfortunately common mistakes by psychotherapists. During the confrontation, a co-therapy team has the practical advantage of reinforcing each other's diagnosis in the face of the patient's denial. They can share the difficult job of reporting the offender and keeping him or her in treatment. If the treatment has been in family therapy, and both therapists judge that mode inappropriate in light of the new information, one of the co-therapists can take the patient into individual treatment while the other can continue work with the family. Many times, the issue of sexual abuse will not emerge until the patient has been treated by co-therapy and the dynamics of the abusive family are thereby stimulated. We speak of this in detail in Chapter 6.

Co-therapists can share major treatment decisions about how to treat and also when not to treat. It is always difficult to deny a patient treatment in a group because he or she is simply not suitable. However, making such a judgment accurately and early in conjunction with one's co-therapist can save many headaches later. As difficult as it is to deny treatment at the initial interview stage, it is even more problematic to terminate treatment once it has begun. This touches on the relatively rare and always burdensome task of asking someone to leave group therapy because he or she is not appropriate for the context of the treatment. Usually, this occurs as a result of a therapist's mistake or misdiagnosis. However, sometimes a group outgrows a certain member after many years as the group itself grows healthier in the aggregate and leaves the particular member far behind. In one such case, we were able to provide another treatment option for the patient. One of us started a group with less functional members and offered it to the patient, thereby mollifying the sense of rejection felt by him.

One practical consequence of co-therapy is increased cost for patients. Employing two therapists for 1 hour or 1 1/2 hours obviously costs more. Because co-therapists do not in most cases double the cost for the therapy hour, therapists earn less per unit of time than they would in solo practice. In private practice, a therapist must be willing to forego as much as 50% of his or her hourly fee in order to practice co-therapy. Many therapists who enjoy co-therapy would probably practice it more, except that it means charging their patients more per hour and receiving less remuneration themselves for each hour they spend.

The utilization of time is also an economic factor. In an institutional setting, the practice of co-therapy is clearly more labor intensive in the treatment of individual patients. For most institutions the choice of co-therapy in individual treatment is not economically wise. However, the phenomenon is more complex than it appears. As the group psychotherapy program at Group Health Cooperative of Puget Sound discovered, co-therapy in the service of group psychotherapy treatment actually proved more economical for two reasons. First, group psychotherapy itself is much less labor intensive than other modes of treatment, and second, co-therapy provided a powerful incentive for therapists to produce more treatment groups.

The desire to co-lead psychotherapy groups produced fortunate results for the group psychotherapy program at Group Health Cooperative. In 1980, the program began to utilize co-therapy teams in the rotational leadership of couples' groups to address a specific problem. The problem was a backlog of referrals for couples' groups and no definite schedule for when new groups would begin. Under this plan, a co-therapy team conducted a couple's group for 8 weeks. At termination of the group, one partner of the team dropped out to be replaced by another therapist. A new 8 week group began, and at its close the member of the original co-therapy dyad, who by then had served 16 weeks in two groups, dropped out, to be replaced by a third therapist who began a new couples' group, and so forth. Rotating co-therapy teams provided continuity in group leadership from one group to the next. It allowed timely planning by the group psychotherapy program and gave referring therapists the certain knowledge that a couples' group was always either in progress or in formation.

Therapists in our survey expressed the belief that therapy itself moves faster by the practice of co-therapy because resistance and anxiety in the patients can be worked through more quickly. Also, each can pace him- or herself more effectively when engaged in co-therapy. Co-therapists can check each other's timing of events. This is of particular import in family or group therapy, when impatience by therapists can disrupt the emergence of process in the treatment setting.

However, co-therapists must overcome difficulties in scheduling appointments. Scheduling individual and family appointments at times possible for two therapists complicates the picture. A lot more co-therapy might be done except that it conflicts with the busy practices of private clinicians. Two therapists may prove compatible in every way except that their schedules do not match. This means that the therapist who wants to practice co-therapy with another clinician must constantly check that person's schedule in order to keep time available in his or her own calendar. This kind of monitoring requires time and effort.

Co-therapists must spend time to develop and maintain their relationship. The expenditure of emotional energy to support the relationship can be quite rewarding. However, overinvolvement with a co-therapist can prove to be an energy drain and an extravagant expenditure of time. Sexual involvements come under this particular caveat, yet nonsexual attachments may also inflict stress on co-therapists. For example, problems may ensue if a co-therapist develops a serious emotional or physical problem. If a co-therapist loses a spouse through divorce or death, his or her partner may be expected to go through that loss as part of relationship maintenance.

### Practical Aspects of Complementarity

Rosenbaum believes that co-therapy teams are best constructed on a symmetrical basis. This means that equality between co-therapists, which he defines as "same type of behavior," takes precedence over complementary behavior in their working relationships. By complementary behavior he means that co-therapists perform different types of functions. He believes this invariably leads to inequality. He states, "An effective co-therapy team works on a symmetrical pattern. Some teams may work effectively in complementary fashion, but their goals appear to be more limited, since one therapist dominates the other" (Rosenbaum, 1983, p. 170). Although the emphasis on equality is well placed, the slighting of the significance of complementarity among effective teams and the belief that it necessarily leads to dominance by one therapist are mistaken. First, equality does not mean doing the "same type of behavior." It means sharing power in the consultative and decision-making processes of therapy. Second, only when persons unequal in knowledge and experience are paired for educational purposes does complementary behavior necessarily imply a hierarchy (see Chapter 2). In such cases, the supervising therapist is the dominant force. However, this is not co-therapy as we define it.

An egalitarian relationship does not preclude complementarity. A truly equal relationship permits a deeper appreciation and acceptance of differences between co-therapists. Such a relationship, in turn, helps clients develop their own capacity for differentiation. The sharing of skills by mature individuals is the highest form of complementarity and in no way compromises the egalitarian structure of their relationship.

There is no better place to illustrate how co-therapy complementarity works than in the realm of practical considerations. It makes good sense to encourage the recognition of differences at this level. For example, in the context of private practice, one person may be much better at marketing the team and thereby stimulate referrals for treatment. He or she may have superior skills in advertising and be quite comfortable with extemporaneous speaking on radio and television— all of which serve to bring people in the door. He or she may also have extensive professional affiliations in hospitals, treatment centers or training institutions that can facilitate a flow of referrals. The other person, however, may be much better at interviewing clients, enlisting their trust, and establishing a bond in the early stages of therapy. He or she can form an early alliance with patients and persuade them to enter a group or begin a course of family therapy. In this way, the essential but different tasks of generating consumer interest and obtaining patient commitment are effectively balanced.

In another example of complementary pairing, one person may produce great ideas and see the big picture of psychotherapy. In private practice, this person might be an entrepreneur and envision plans for ambitious ventures. On the other hand, his or her partner may be much better at the actual business of psychotherapy and better at putting plans into action. He or she may have a good memory for details, be proficient with statistics and the intricacies of billing patients, and possess other key management and organizational skills. From such a fortuitous match, a co-therapy team can thrive and prosper.

Other complementary skills include the ability to write about one's clinical experiences and the ability to edit those writings; the ability to remain optimistic during the difficult process of starting a therapy group and the ability to be realistic about the number of people needed to begin; the ability to handle phone calls well as part of the initial process of interviewing patients and the capacity to be inviting and accepting in the first face-to-face meeting with them.

Also, the kind of clients that each member of the co-therapy team attracts will vary, based on the drawing power of each individual personality. A co-therapist with different family-of-origin issues than oneself will probably have divergent professional interests and, therefore, appeal to a different clientele. For example, the co-therapist with a personal history of bulimia may have greater success in recruiting patients for an eating disorder group because of the patients' identification with him or her.

## THE SPECIFIC NATURE OF THE CO-THERAPY RELATIONSHIP

Earlier in this chapter we discussed those dimensions of the co-therapy relationship that had treatment consequences and how those consequences are frequently given as reasons for choosing the practice of co-therapy. Whereas the specific nature of the co-therapy relationship also has treatment consequences, the relationship itself is a characteristic of the co-therapy practice and not the primary reason for selecting co-therapy. The co-therapy relationship can evolve from friends, colleagues, lovers, marriage partners, business associates, or combinations thereof. Such relationships can express a wide degree of comfort with professional intimacy and closeness or distance.

When two persons contract to be co-therapists, they may be strangers curious about the prospect of getting to know each other better, or they may be friends or perhaps colleagues who have a history with each other in many contexts. They may be lovers or marriage partners who wish to explore their ability to work together and share professional responsibilities. Or they may be two persons who, as a result of working together as co-therapists, choose to become lovers. In this case, the disclosure or nondisclosure of their union presents special problems for them and their patients. They simply may be business associates who want to share each others' skills and agree to share a task of importance to both. For each team, the reasons why they initially joined forces, the specific nature of their relationship, and the boundaries they establish for themselves within their relationship will circumscribe what they can accomplish in the psychotherapy.

Strangers may grow in their admiration and trust of each other and, given enough time practicing co-therapy, may choose to become friends or colleagues. Others may choose to stop their mutual work, whether from lack of satisfaction with the arrangement or from lack of results with their patients. Either way, much time will be devoted to defining the co-therapy relationship at the beginning, and consequently, the therapy pair will simply not be as attentive or watchful of their clients during this early period. They will be watching each other instead.

The prospect of needing time at the beginning to establish a working contract is not unique to strangers. Friends and colleagues must also devote time at the beginning to surmount the many challenges faced in the early phases of the co-therapy relationship. Jim Dugo and Ariadne Beck discuss this in detail in Chapter 7. It is our belief that friends and colleagues may pass through these phases quicker than strangers and thereby be available to clients as a team sooner. However, there is no guarantee that it will happen that way. Entering into a co-therapy arrangement has a way of arousing questions we have about ourselves and exposing vulnerabilities and fears that are otherwise kept well defended and hidden.

Max Rosenbaum has cogently remarked on this phenomenon:

> The group therapist who has successfully masked omnipotent behavior, a need to be seductive, a need to avoid anger, or a need to stimulate hostility will almost certainly have his behavior and needs exposed when another therapist joins the group. Of course, the therapist with problems of omniscience may select as a co-therapist someone who will not rock the boat. (1983, p. 170)

Lovers and marriage partners are not exempt from the necessary discovery process at the start of co-therapy. In fact, their bonds may be highly vulnerable if their motivations for being together have not been thoroughly examined prior to co-therapy. Co-therapy itself can prove to be a hazard to relationships, as we discuss at length in Chapter 5. However, if the couple relationship has a firm foundation, it may provide a base for complementary interaction. Each person can draw on a loving atmosphere within the family. The couple's skill in managing conflict at home will prove helpful as arguments and differences surface in their work together. The style of communication that they have created will clearly show in their collaboration as co-therapists.

The specific characteristics of the co-therapy team include not only the nature of the relationship but also the degree of psychological intimacy they share and the depth of knowledge they have about each other. On this dimension, some friends may enjoy greater intimacy than some marriage partners. To that extent, their ease and facility working together may prove far superior to that of a married team. The conflicts that emerge in the treatment of patients are sure to test the sufficiency of the resolutions and compromises made by husband-and-wife teams. A willingness to share self-knowledge is another factor that can vary across the many possible co-therapy combinations. It may be easier for some people to share their self-doubts with strangers than with people they have known for years.

All these factors limit what a given team can accomplish by their co-therapy. The degree of comfort each team experiences with professional closeness or distance sets a limit on how far its co-therapy relationship will develop. In Chapter 7, Dugo and Beck detail precisely what a co-therapy team can accomplish in group psychotherapy as it progresses along the first three phases of co-therapy team development. They propose a developmental framework in which certain tasks must be accomplished by the co-therapists at each phase. From this we can deduce that, for example, a team in the later phases of co-therapy development that has accomplished the task of interdependence will provide more objective and accurate feedback to their group and themselves than the team in an earlier phase that is dependent on each other and insulates itself from all sources of criticism. For any co-therapy pair, the opportunity to go deeper into the self is always there, as well as the chance to explore how the self can relate with another. This is clearly a choice that many therapists relish. Whatever the specific nature of the co-therapy team, it is clear that therapists are choosing not only a special practice of psychotherapy but also a relationship. The specific nature of that relationship contains unique possiblities for therapeutic interactions with patients.

Co-therapy can provide much joy, excitement, and stimulation for therapists. The sheer joy of working together at a worthwhile task is laudable. Creativity and problem solving can be a source of mutual stimulation. Friendship and comradeship can reward co-therapists richly for the many hours they spend together. The shared excitement of seeing a patient change over time can deepen the meaning of the therapeutic encounter.

The nature of the co-therapy relationship can also be a sexual one.*

---

*The sexual attraction between male and female co-leaders of group psychotherapy has been the subject of a study by Eleanor White, RN, PhD. She believes

This is obvious in the case of husband-and-wife teams. However, some co-therapists are committed to each other in heterosexual or homosexual relationships without marriage and let their clients know about their commitment. Clients use this knowledge of intimacy in many ways. Some choose to forget about it entirely, whereas others imagine their co-therapists as a perfect or idyllic couple. However the clients respond, it usually indicates some therapeutic issue for them that can be dealt with openly in the therapy.

Where the co-therapists are single or committed to others, clients still fantasize about romantic connections between the co-therapists, and this may or may not emerge as a topic for therapy. When the co-therapists are involved sexually and find it is more convenient, desirable, or necessary from their point of view to keep their sexual liaisons a secret, clients cannot discuss their fantasies and have no venue in which to discuss their suspicions. Clients are highly adaptive and will not bring up material that the therapists want to remain secret.

It is our belief that when the sexual activity of the co-therapy team is implicitly denied or omitted from the knowledge of the patients and/or co-workers in the treatment setting, the co-therapy team is inviting trouble. At best, such a secret can lead to personal confusion or co-worker suspicion. At worst, it can lead to massive denial, deception, and acting out in the treatment room and dismissal or resignation from the workplace. The case where sexual activity is intentionally kept secret is discussed in detail in Chapter 5. The case where sexual involvement is open knowledge or a marital couple forms a co-therapy team is discussed below.

### The Openly Sexual Co-Therapy Relationship

Co-therapists who are married or otherwise committed to each other in relationships that are both intimate and sexual portray a special picture to the patients they treat. Here is a couple that not only respects each other and shares tasks equally but also sleeps together. This becomes a powerful image in the minds of the couple's clients.

Open sexual involvement between co-therapists can certainly heighten the intensity of the transference between patients and therapists. For example, when patients in a group are focusing on teenage issues in which sexual identity and expression become paramount, they are keenly aware that they can learn from the co-therapy couple

---

that heightened sexual attraction between co-therapists has consequences for both the co-therapy team and the group and that the phenomenon is more common than recognized in the literature.

who makes their sexual relationship known. Married co-therapists are able to do that. So are co-therapists who are committed to each other as a couple. In these cases, openness of the sexual involvement can become a part of the treatment process. How does that happen?

During Phase IV of Ariadne Beck's (1981b) theory of the development of psychotherapy groups, discussions of intimacy and closeness emerge (see Appendix). Coping with sexuality in personal relationships becomes a major theme. At the level of the group, expressions of tenderness and closeness to each other will flourish, and there will be room for playfulness among members. Fantasies about the group and its members will be raised openly and accepted as appropriate topics for discussion. At the level of the individual, several issues will emerge. Sexuality as it affects any relationship must be faced. "How will I manage my sexual responses to others in group?" becomes a major concern. Group members will experiment with various ways to express their tenderness and caring for each other. They will demonstrate trust for each other as they establish the ground rules for intimacy in their group.

During this phase, the co-therapy team must come across more as people than as authorities. A married co-therapy team can move confidently and comfortably in the realm of sexual relations and sexual feelings and can help the group discover its emotional process around these issues. If the co-therapy team is willing and it is appropriate, it can describe the subtle dimensions of the sexually intimate relationship: the fear of loss, the anguish of jealousy, the wish to possess, the temptation to dominate, the necessity to compromise for the sake of mutual desire, the joy of sexual fulfillment, the gratification of the need to be loved, and the pleasure of loving companionship. This becomes an especially rich period in the life of the psychotherapy group and prepares the group emotionally so it can confront the difficult issues of dependency and hostility in the next phase of group development.

Like any co-therapy team, married therapists must resolve the issues of erotic transference and power (Golden & Golden, 1976). On these issues, the married team is ahead in several ways. First, they have already established their sexual boundaries. Whereas the unmarried co-therapy pair must attend to that task (see Phase 1 of co-therapy team development in Chapter 7) and generally excludes the co-worker as a sexual partner, the married pair has accomplished it and generally includes the other as a sexual partner. Second, their sexual knowledge of each other lends credibility to what they say about sexuality. A patient can trust that they have experienced a range of emotions in their relations with each other. For example, in couple therapy, a male therapist can discuss with the husband the manifold feelings brought on by occasional impotency in the marriage bed. Their discussion can be especially frank and empathic and have a healing effect for the marriage.

Third, if the relationship is healthy and mature, the modeling of touch and self-disclosure can be easier. The demonstration of physical touch and the sharing of how the therapist couple has confronted and overcome similar problems can be powerful ways to surmount resistance of clients to change. This clinical approach has been especially relevant in the treatment of couples for sexual dysfunction and in the treatment of couples in general. Couples learn how to tackle their problems, and they see before them an example of at least moderate success.

Although not referring to married co-therapists specifically, William Masters and Virginia Johnson believed "a more successful clinical approach to problems of sexual dysfunction can be made by dual-sex teams of therapists than by an individual male or female therapist" (1970, p. 4). It was their assertion that dual-sex teams provide sexual allies for the same-sex clients and sexual translators for the opposite-sex clients. Other clinicians have challenged their claims in the area of treating sexual dyfunction (Zilbergeld & Evans, 1980). LoPiccolo, Heiman, Hogan, and Roberts (1985) offer an informative outcome study on this topic, but there is a telling omission that unfortunately is characterisic of outcome studies in this field. That omission is the failure to understand the importance of employing experienced co-therapy teams in the application of co-therapy. The authors say their therapists vary in experience but give no indication of how long or in what depth each co-therapy team has worked together. Their study appraised only one of three variables that must be considered, the dual sex of the co-therapy team. But it did not address two other variables: (1) the length of time working together and to what depth and (2) whether the co-therapists are married. These variables might give a different picture if studied independently as factors in the treatment of couples.

Our own survey also neglected to ask "How long have you worked with a particular therapist in a co-therapy team?" In this way we have followed a standard pattern of investigators in the field who have overlooked this as an important variable.

The struggle for power can prove to be an obstacle for married co-therapists. Unless the desire to dominate has been sublimated or in some way controlled, it will sabotage treatment goals. In that case, the great familiarity of married co-therapy teams, instead of being a strong base for effective communication, can become a source of ammunition for partners bent on exposing their companions' vulnerabilities. Married partners who work together must learn to delight in the power the other manifests. This is a different understanding of the concept of power. It is the power to make known and not the power to control. It is a joy to be able to brag about one's co-worker. This has been especially true for us as co-therapists and marriage partners. The experience of watching each other competently handle a formidable clinical task has enriched our lives and deepened our appreciation for one another as people and professionals. The pleasure displayed by the co-therapy couple can be very exciting for patients to see as a model of what is possible in a marriage. Co-therapy can be an on-going stimulus for the growth of the marriage when this level of functioning has been achieved.

A married couple must not, however, take for granted that their special knowledge of each other guarantees an easy transition to co-therapy. They must plan and organize their work together in a disciplined fashion, just as they would with any other professional relationship. The emphasis on professionalism is quite pertinent. There is no room for casualness in preparation or evaluation because it will lead to less than satisfactory results for their clients and perhaps even lead to blaming and disputes in their relationship where none had existed before.

### The Unequal Team

Married therapists who are not equally competent and knowledgeable as therapists face all the problems encountered by any therapist and assistant therapist pairing—and more. We believe their collaboration is a fraudulent contract unless both parties acknowledge the inequality to their patients and establish a plan whereby the assistant therapist can learn and grow. It is highly advisable for such a team to consult with a trusted and experienced therapist as a third party to supervise and mediate their efforts to co-lead. Such a plan is both clinically astute and emotionally healthy for the marriage. Otherwise, many dilemmas can complicate the treatment and training process. The accomplished therapist in the pair may allow mistakes to go uncorrected in an effort to be kind or patronizing. The therapist, out of jealousy, may not allow the assistant therapist to grow toward equality. The assistant therapist may take offense at the constructive criticism of the spouse, regardless of how tactfully it is presented. Unnoticed feelings of inadequacy or competitiveness may erupt suddenly in the context of treatment. Without a third party to supervise, any of the above occurrences can threaten the therapy or the marriage or both. We talk more about the special problems of spouses or lovers who are bona fide co-therapists in Chapter 5.

We have considered in depth the case where psychotherapists who are equals become co-therapy teams. What happens when therapists who are not equal, or when peers who are not fully trained therapists, form dyads? This is the subject we discuss in the next chapter.

# • 2 •

# *Educational Reasons for Shared Leadership*

Over 40 years ago, Hadden (1947) advocated a method of teaching psychotherapy in which a "junior therapist" joined a "colleague" in a group treatment setting. This method was considered salutory because it permitted the less experienced therapist to observe the therapist and receive feedback.

In 1974, Dies polled practicing group psychotherapists on their opinions about the utility of various training methods. "Co-therapy experience with a qualified therapist" was chosen by them as the most helpful training experience. "Co-therapy experience with a peer, followed by sessions with a supervisor" placed fourth among their preferences. The results of another survey (Dies, 1980) showed that 27 out of 100 supervisors who were experienced in the training of group psychotherapists advocated co-therapy as a training method for group psychotherapy.

Our survey corroborated the popularity of such training methods among group therapists. Seventy of 80 therapists who responded to the question, "Will you or would you do co-therapy with a person who is in training with you or under your supervision?" replied affirmatively.

Clearly the organization of supervisor–trainee and trainee–trainee dyads in order to enhance the learning of students of psychotherapy is common practice and firmly entrenched. However, we do not consider pairings for educational purposes to be co-therapy.

## SPECIAL DEFINITIONS FOR UNEQUAL AND NON-THERAPIST TEAMS

The supervisor–trainee relationship is not co-therapy because it is not *equal*, and the trainee–trainee relationship is not co-therapy because neither is a *therapist*.★ The term co-therapist is neither accurate nor satisfactory when applied to either pair. Yet such teams are common in the training of therapists and so must have names.

We propose special terminology to designate leadership pairs who are not, in fact, co-therapists but who work together for the purpose of education. Two students who undertake a mode of therapy together under the aegis of a supervisor we call *co-learners* because they are equal in experience and knowledge and both are learning the process of therapy. Together they co-learn in the context of group, family, or individual therapy. We do not want to imply by this that students of therapy do less-than-adequate work. We simply want to indicate that they are not fully trained therapists and so, by definition, cannot be co-therapists. On the other hand, a supervisor and a student or a therapist and an assistant therapist who undertake a mode of therapy together we call *nequipos* (pronounced ně kwĭ′ pōs). We call them nequipos because they are neither equal in experience nor equally equipped with the knowledge and authority to do therapy. The root word is *equipo*, which is Spanish and means "team." Together they constitute an unequal team in the context of group, family, or individual therapy.

We propose the terms co-learners and nequipos to help clarify these popular training methods and distinguish them from co-therapy. Psychotherapists learn much from co-therapy, but treatment, not learning, is the primary goal. Students and supervisors help patients as co-learners and nequipos, but learning has equal standing with treatment as a major goal.

A nequipo team cannot practice co-therapy as we define it, since it is not a relationship between peers. It does not presume an equality of knowledge, experience, or skills. One person is a therapist and teacher, and the other is an assistant therapist and trainee. It is an arrangement in

★There is an important exception to this statement that involves the case of a therapist being paired with a non-therapist for educational reasons. An example is the team in which an experienced therapist returning for postgraduate education joins a graduate student without clinical experience. The supervisor of their work together must establish a contract similar to that for co-learners, but one that takes into account the unequal experience of the students.

which most of the learning goes in one direction. There is not the expectation of a mutual exchange, although over time an assistant therapist may perform skills at peer capacity with his or her teacher. We designed a questionnaire for selecting co-therapists, and we recommend that it also be applied in the pairing of nequipos (see Chapter 3). The therapist must be willing to match his or her responses to the questionnaire with those of the assistant therapist. Because the therapist holds major decision-making power, we recommend that he or she initiate a dialogue with the assistant therapist adapting the exercises we suggest to the kind of nequipo team he or she wants to create (see Chapter 3).

Over the short term, less than 6 months, the use of nequipos remains a teaching method of uncertain value. What usefulness it has surely does not derive from the relationship between the nequipos. Learning by way of videotapes, seminars, and experiential workshops would probably be as rich. Over the long term, 6 months to 3 years, the relationship between nequipos can produce significant teaching value. Our minimum definition for a long-term contract is 24 hours contact time in treatment sessions and 12 hours contact time for post-treatment discussion and feedback. We think of this contract in terms of 6 months, during which 1 hour treatment sessions occur each week followed by 1/2 hour post-treatment discussion, but a different configuration of hours could satisfy this minimal standard. The nequipos' value to their patients also will increase as the inequality between them diminishes and their budding co-therapy relationship begins to mature. In the case of nequipos, we recommend a teaching method that is close to the mentor-protege model in which both commit to a master-apprenticeship contract for a number of years.

The co-learner arrangement also does not constitute co-therapy. Although the students are peers, they are still not therapists. Over the short term, the use of co-learners has no greater value as a training method than nequipos, although Yalom (1970) believes that the method has special advantages for the beginning therapist. Whereas it is true that co-learners may be able to help each other differentiate between what is real and what is transference distortion in the patients' perceptions, their ability to do so depends on the availability of an astute supervisor, the quality of his or her feedback, and the maturity of the co-learners as clinicians and as a dyad. The pairing of co-learners for less than 6 months will not allow them to evolve as a team beyond the earliest phases of development, and this will limit what they are able to learn from each other and restrict what they can accomplish clinically. In the short term co-learners will benefit most from ob serving someone at the same level of professional development as themselves. This kind of identification, although not a substitute for a working relationship, can provide succor for anxious trainees.

We suspect that the choice of the co-learner method of training is too often a matter of convenience. A supervisor wants two students exposed to group therapy, and there are only enough referrals for one group. Or a supervisor wants two students involved in family therapy but has time only to observe work with one family by tapes or one-way mirror. Such reasons are not sufficient for employing co-learners. However expedient or convenient such a practice may be for a training institution, it is important to remember that the pairing of therapists, including student therapists, *always* has treatment consequences. The supervisor must consider the time commitment necessary in order to train co-learners, and that commitment must include an on-going analysis of their developing relationship.

## CO-THERAPY RESEARCH WITH CO-LEARNERS, NEQUIPOS, AND NOVICE CO-THERAPISTS

Most research in the field of co-therapy does not study fully functioning co-therapy teams (Kosch & Reiner, 1983; LoPiccolo, et al, 1985; Piper, Doan, Edwards, & Jones, 1979; Roman & Meltzer, 1977). Many studies neglect to mention an all-important variable: how long the teams under study have worked together. Other studies investigate teams that appear to have worked together less than 5 months. One half year is not much time according to authors who have described phases of co-therapy development (Dick, Lessler, & Whiteside, 1980; Hoffman & Hoffman, 1981; Winter, 1976). It is hardly enough time to complete the second phase of co-therapy development according to Dugo and Beck's model (Chapter 7). Such teams have just confronted the strong, competitive urges that test their commitment and are only just beginning to function as a cooperative unit. Employing therapists who are inexperienced in the practice of co-therapy with each other in order to study the effectiveness of co-therapy is simply misguided. It shows a deep misunderstanding of the co-therapy enterprise. In such research, co-therapy is not being examined at all. Rather, the difficulty of two strangers relating to each other in an unfamiliar setting is being studied.

Employing co-learners and nequipos as research subjects is also a mistaken practice if these teams have not been working together for at least a year. If they are co-learners, they are peers, but equality of inexperience and fear will not generate any meaningful data on co-leadership. If they are nequipos, they must attain some operational parity before they will be able to give an approximate account of what co-therapy can accomplish.

Co-therapy teams are developed. They do not spring fully formed into the therapeutic milieu. Time is needed. Concentration and hard work and listening are required in the early months and years of a developing relationship. A few of the milestones that must be passed in the progress of a team are presented in Chapter 7. Co-therapists must know more than therapists, and more is required of them than of solo therapists. Further research in the field should be conducted with subjects who are experienced both in psychotherapy and as co-therapists in order to produce data that carry greater meaning for the clinician.

## RULES FOR SUPERVISORS

In the training situation, where nequipos have committed to a year or more of learning in the context of psychotherapy practice, the therapist must take greater responsibility for the way their relationship develops. However, taking greater responsibility for the relationship does not imply dominating the therapy. We agree with Bernard, Babineau, and Schwartz (1980) that the trainee must be accorded time to initiate his or her interventions as often as possible. The paradoxical permission, "Make as many mistakes as you can," is helpful. The student will focus on what he or she must learn to become a psychotherapist. It is too much to expect the student to observe the co-therapy relationship simply because there are too many things happening that must be grasped first. It is the therapist's job to monitor their relationship to be sure it is not impeding learning objectives or the treatment process. If it is, then this method of teaching should be modified or terminated.

In like fashion, the supervisor of co-learners must also bear major responsibility for what is happening or not happening between the two students. Again, the co-learners' primary focus will be on the therapy situation and the clients. The supervisor must introduce the factor of the co-therapy relationship and observe closely its progress.

The therapist or supervisor can always question his or her student therapists to see if their needs are being met. But realistically, many students will not be aware of their needs in a relationship to a master therapist. They may be too much involved in pleasing the master therapist or competing for strokes or building their sense of personal adequacy and professional competence or being afraid.

If a therapist intends to teach from the nequipo position or if a supervisor intends to supervise co-learners, he or she must be prepared to spell out for students how the co-therapy relationship can work and how it should look. It's a double job for the therapists: (1) teach the student and (2) monitor the relationship. The nequipo and co-learner relationships will not take care of themselves. They will need attention, especially in the early phases; should they not receive attention, they can and will undermine the best teaching.

Because the student must form a complicated relationship as a condition for this training method, the method itself can easily become an obstacle to the training. The following rules are designed to help avoid common problems.

### Specific Rules for Therapists in Nequipo Teams

1. Establish a learning contract that clearly distinguishes this training experience from co-therapy.
2. Provide a theoretical model of how co-therapy teams evolve. Dugo and Beck provide one such model in Chapter 7.
3. Encourage questions, especially naive ones and those that challenge your own theories and practices.
4. Express congruence. Be frank about what you know and what you don't know.
5. Formulate questions yourself and communicate your sense of curiosity.
6. Anticipate the student's questions and dilemmas.
7. Acknowledge and support the student's growing sense of beginning competence.
8. Eschew one-upsmanship and unnecessary competition.
9. Share with your student your own fears in the present and those you felt as a trainee.
10. Observe and listen to the student closely, and generously acknowledge what you learn from him or her.

### Specific Rules for Supervisors of Co-Learners

1. Follow the rules that apply to nequipos.
2. Discourage competition among co-learners for your approval.
3. Acknowledge co-learners equally and recognize the different strengths each brings to the treatment setting.
4. Let them know that they can deepen their work affiliation if they choose to do so.

5. Encourage open and direct communication. As a safeguard, meet with each of the co-learners separately at least once during the course of supervision so that co-learners can speak frankly about their relationship.

Most of these principles apply to all successful co-therapy situations, as we describe further in Chapter 4. But in the training context of co-learners and nequipos, it is paramount that the therapist or supervisor take the greater share of responsibility, foreseeing difficulties and solving problems creatively. If the therapist or supervisor is unwilling or unable to make such a commitment of time and effort, he or she should not train from the nequipo position or supervise co-learners. The nature of this sort of training puts greater demands on the therapist.

## THE LEARNING CONTRACT

A learning contract should be drawn up between nequipos. (See Appendix for an example of such a contract.) Goals for the assistant therapist should be clarified and agreed on by the therapist. Also, the therapist must specify the responsibilities that he or she expects the assistant therapist to assume. Learning is advanced significantly when a trainee can watch and imitate the style of a competent therapist. The therapist must encourage the therapeutic assertiveness of the trainee and do so in a nonpatronizing way. One of the ways to encourage therapeutic assertiveness is to plan for the assistant therapist to conduct several sessions alone. This will help the assistant therapist grow in confidence (Alpher & Kobos, 1988). If the therapist is also supervising the assistant therapist in a training program that grades performance or an internship that monitors hours of experience, the therapist must watch especially for signs of dependency and overcompliance in his or her assistant therapist. The therapist must clarify his or her own therapeutic strategies by verbalizing what he or she is doing. Remember, it is not the primary goal of most therapists to teach the skills of co-therapy. Rather, their goal is to teach the skills of therapy. The method of teaching they employ is based on such a complex relationship that the following conditions must be addressed in the learning contract; the failure to do so may lead to an abuse of the relationship between nequipos.

The therapist must inform the assistant therapist of the difficulties and problems inherent in the nequipo training method and invite his or her discussion of these matters. The assistant therapist should know that he or she may be scapegoated by the patients, and a strategy should be devised to address its possible occurrence. If the training fails, the therapist must not blame the student. This is another kind of scape-goating and can be avoided by a proper understanding of the limita-tions of the method and the risks involved. The therapist must know how he or she will profit by the training arrangement and make that clear to the assistant therapist. If this involves the assistant therapist paying the therapist, this arrangement should be spelled out in the contract. Nequipos must avoid the situation where the assistant ther-apist simply gratifies the therapist as an audience for his or her brilliant maneuvers. The therapist must also inform patients that they are being treated by a nequipo team.

Some authors have stressed the time commitment entailed by co-therapy (Dick et al., 1980). This holds true for the training situation. Adequate training programs must consider 1 to 3 years as realistic time periods for nequipos to become functioning co-therapy teams. Learning contracts between nequipos of less than 1/2 year we consider unadvisable because of possible harm to the assistant therapist and loss of benefit to the patients. Given the conditions of commitment and time, the teaching can be excellent, since so much rich and immediate data are available for analysis by nequipos.

A learning contract should also be drawn up between co-learners and their supervisors. (See Appendix for an example of such a con-tract.) The goals for the students should be clarified and agreed on. In the establishment of a learning contract, the supervisor should invite assertiveness on the part of the students and thereby set the tone for the training experience that follows. The supervisor should advocate a contract that helps the students grow in confidence and autonomy as clinicians. As is true in the case of nequipos, the primary goal of those who supervise co-learners is to teach them the skills of therapy. How-ever, the method of teaching that a supervisor employs with co-learners is complicated. The supervisor must be aware of the specific relationship that develops between co-learners and how their relation-ship can impede learning as well as the therapy. The supervisor must also be aware of the transferential implications of his or her relationship with each student. Will he or she supervise as a distant authority, or will he or she be more available as a person? The supervisor should let the students know his or her preferred style beforehand.

The supervisor must also advise co-learners of the difficulties and problems inherent to the co-learning method and invite their discus-sion of these matters. For example, competition can overwhelm the efforts of co-learners to collaborate in the psychotherapy. The super-visor must be aware of the competition going on between co-learners and help them attain a level of communication that allows them to function cooperatively. Whereas the chief obstacle in nequipo training is scapegoating, the chief obstacle in co-learner training is uncontrolled competition. It is the supervisor's job to monitor this phenomenon. The supervisor must also instruct co-learners to inform clients that they are therapists in training.

Co-learners fear making mistakes. Either one or both may have a tendency to hold back his or her interventions, thereby assuming too passive a stance in the psychotherapy. The supervisor must encourage the therapeutic assertiveness of co-learners and help them see the importance of taking risks in the service of learning therapy. Giving examples from one's own clinical practice, and especially mistakes, helps the students to incorporate the trial-and-error method into their repertoire.

If the co-learners have not had the opportunity to choose their partner, or if sufficient time has not been spent in the process of selection, co-learners may be resentful of the co-learning pair in which they find themselves. For this reason we recommend, whenever possible, that co-learners be given the opportunity to choose their partners. Supervisors should provide prospective co-learners with practical instruments and exercises designed to assist in the selection process similar to those we provide for co-therapists in Chapter 3.

We want to reiterate that training programs must consider 1 to 3 years as realistic time periods for co-learners to become fully functioning co-therapy teams. Learning contracts between supervisors and co-learners of less than 1/2 year we consider unadvisable because of the possible harm to the co-learners and loss of benefit to the clients. Clients experience a double loss in short-term treatment by co-learner dyads. They lose because no therapist is directly involved in their treatment, and they lose again because the co-learners have not had time to become a functional team. Co-learners may blame each other or experience a sense of failure in the treatment of their patients if they do not have adequate time to resolve conflicts in their relationship. They may postulate from their negative experience that group or family therapy is not for them.

Because there are many reasons why a co-learner pair may not work out, the learning contract should specify that the members end their association without having to assume a sense of failure. Training from the co-learning position entails many risks, and one of these risks is the possibility of an inappropriate match of co-learners. Supervisors should be aware of this possibility, and, rather than persist with an unfortunate co-learner association, they should be able to see the error and be willing to terminate the contract. Damage to either co-learners, their patients, or both may ensue if such a procedure is not followed.

The supervisor must make clear to co-learners the specific reasons why he or she has chosen to teach from a co-learner position and what personal payback the supervisor will obtain. If the supervisor works for an organization, is this kind of training required by custom or job regulation? Will he or she be paid for the supervision, and if so, by whom? If the state law permits the co-learners to pay the supervisor directly for the training experience, they especially have a right to ask if co-learning is the most beneficial kind of training for them and why the supervisor believes this to be so.

Some authors have experienced good luck using the nequipo training method in the context of individual treatment (Bernard et al. 1980). They report that advanced students possess enough therapy skills to profit from the more sophisticated therapeutic strategies of the therapists. Students who are novices, however, must confine themselves to learning how to form a therapeutic alliance with a patient. In this particular training program, supervisory sessions from 1/2 hour to 1 hour in length take place immediately after treatment sessions. Such post-treatment sessions are a good practice and should be considered in the learning contract.

The kind of learning and feedback that co-therapy provides is welcome to therapists at any level of competence. Rosenbaum (1977) states, "Even experienced psychotherapists learn from the practice of co-therapy." In the field of group psychotherapy, the gulf between the novice therapist and the experienced therapist is not so great as some imagine. The practice of group psychotherapy challenges even the most capable group therapist. Everyone must practice with a measure of uncertainty and humility. There are masters of group therapy, but there are no experts (Roller, 1984).

## NEQUIPO TEAMS IN ACTION

Nequipo teams are so prevalent that they deserve special attention in order to understand their operation. The following are vignettes of how such teams behave, including some of the rewards and pitfalls one can encounter.

### Acknowledging the Assistant Therapist

Wolfgang was a nationally famous family therapist who trained a few selected students and delighted in giving exhibitions of family treatment before professional audiences, employing his students as nequipos for the presentations. At one presentation for the staff of a psychiatric hospital, his student Heidi assisted him in the treatment of a schizophrenic and his family. Wolfgang dominated the presentation by interviewing the parents and making comments to the audience. He appeared wholly absorbed in his work with the family and totally unaware of the presence of his assistant. Forty-five minutes into the therapy hour, Heidi made her first intervention by addressing the youngest sibling who had not uttered a single word. The child, who up to this point had manifested notably agitated behavior, appeared soothed by her comment and grew calm. Heidi followed this with a series of astute observations that succinctly summarized the painful dilemma of the family. The path the family needed to take became clear, and the demonstration came to a close.

The audience seemed puzzled. On the surface this appeared to be an out-of-balance nequipo team. It looked as if Wolfgang did all the "therapy" while Heidi remained inactive. In fact, Heidi had been exercising her formidable power of observation. By her intervention, she had interpreted the anxiety of the youngest child. She was also able to translate verbally the double bind experienced by the identified patient. As the audience applauded, Wolfgang turned and applauded Heidi, graciously acknowledging her contribution. These nequipos were well balanced after all, she as a talented therapist and he as an outstanding teacher.

### An Unacknowledged Nequipo Team

By contrast, another well-known family therapist introduced his wife as his "co-therapist" at the beginning of their demonstration with a group of couples at a national conference. Mrs. Kay said absolutely nothing during the entire hour, while Mr. Kay and all four couples talked loquaciously. The demonstration was designed to give a sense of how the co-therapy team began a couples' group. However, what the audience saw was a highly unbalanced nequipo team. What was most disturbing about this demonstration was the lack of comment by the members of the group regarding the silence of the female "co-therapist." An unacknowledged nequipo team of this sort will prove troubling and even damaging to couples who look to the therapists as models. Mary Goulding gives an example of this in Chapter 8, page 200, and we give another example in Chapter 5, page 118.

### A Seductive Assistant Therapist

Cecelia was a warm and friendly psychiatric nurse who taught group therapy to psychiatric residents at a major medical center. Her preference was to teach from the nequipo position, and she asked Rudolfo to join her in an on-going outpatient adolescent group she had been conducting for 3 years. Rudolfo was a young and handsome first-year psychiatric resident who had come from Europe to study in the United States. At the time Rudolfo entered, the group consisted of eight teenage males and females who acted out their rebellion against parents and other authority figures in socially inappropriate ways. Cecelia wrote a learning contract with Rudolfo specifying that he would lead the group alone three times during the year of his training with her. In the first session Rudolfo surprised Cecelia by complimenting her on her appearance and stroking her hair lightly with his hand. Cecelia said nothing but later in the group she noticed Rudolfo staring intently at her bodice. After the session, she commented on his stare wondering aloud what that was about. Rudolfo said frankly that he was admiring her and that his behavior was simply part of his personality and perfectly acceptable in his culture. Cecelia replied that such behavior was not appropriate in a therapy group, especially when the leaders were in a position to model social norms for teenagers.

Despite subsequent admonitions, Rudolfo continued to exhibit seductive behavior toward his teacher during the group. Cecelia voiced her concern that he was adversely affecting the patients in group and expressed her reservations about allowing him to conduct the group alone as they had planned. Cecelia worried that she might have instigated his flirting by being overly friendly or seductive herself. She suggested that Rudolfo meet with her and another member of the medical school faculty for conjoint supervision, but he refused. When one of the females in group suddenly sat on Rudolfo's lap and coyly remarked, "Look at me the way you do Cecelia," his seductiveness was confirmed. Cecelia insisted on conjoint supervision. During the third-party consultation, Rudolfo revealed his insecurity around women in authority and his need to see them as sexual objects in order to quell his own fears. He agreed to enter psychotherapy to resolve this underlying issue for himself. He admitted that his actions had impacted the group negatively and agreed to continue conjoint supervision. Cecelia was relieved to learn that her responses to Rudolfo had not been inappropriate. After a rocky start, they were able to build a workable nequipo team.

### Collusion with a Patient's Denial

When Bill organizes a nequipo team as a mentor–protege relationship, he does so with the explicit goal of bringing the assistant therapist to a position of relatively equal power, usually within 3 years. However, even the most conscientious nequipos stumble over obstacles on the road to a bona fide co-therapy relationship. Tracy was a talented intern who prevailed on Bill to supervise him in a therapy group from the nequipo position. He had studied group process with Bill and wanted to benefit from intensive clinical work with his teacher. He entered a long-term group that consisted of seven highly functional individuals and one borderline personality, Linda. The group had been in operation for 2 months, and Bill was not certain how the borderline would work out in this context. He was afraid that the presence of the borderline would inhibit the others in their expression of anger, since they perceived Linda as more "fragile" than themselves. Tracy saw Linda in that light also, and she appeared to him as a victim in one of his dreams that was discussed in supervision. Bill saw Linda as a skillful manipulator and was willing to be manipulated if it led to her divulgence of the sexual abuse that she had suffered as a child in her family of origin. However, Linda never revealed her secret in group, and when Tracy and Bill discussed her case months after her departure from group, Bill was surprised to learn that Tracy had been unaware of Bill's perception of her as a manipulator. Differences between nequipos are often perceived as threatening by the assistant therapist who wants to appear competent in the eyes of his mentor and does not want to contradict him. In this way, the nequipo team is at a disadvantage, especially in the early phases of its development, because its sharing is not yet equal, and the mentor does not give the same credence to the assistant therapist's opinions as he will later. Bill did not want to overwhelm Tracy's difference of perception and so did not debate the issue of victim versus manipulator that in a co-therapy team might have led to a powerful intervention: "Linda, Tracy sees you as a victim, and I see you as a manipulator. Tell the group what happened to you in your family so that you became both a victim and a manipulator." Such an intervention would have broken the denial of sexual abuse that ultimately engulfed the group.

Instead, the nequipos colluded with Linda's denial by encouraging her to "take her time" in exposing her secrets to the group. It was as if time itself would become the agent of healing, and this became the group illusion as they repeated the denial in the family of origin. The nequipos mistakenly believed that trust would increase with time, whereas the opposite was true. The trust of the borderline patient would have increased with confrontation. Tracy and Bill confronted the group about their lack of anger, and yet they themselves avoided confronting Linda about her abuse, which would have brought forth her rage. The nequipos projected their own avoidance of anger onto the group.

### Training a Family Practice Resident

The Family Practice Residency of a large health maintenance organization, in conjunction with the Mental Health Service, instituted a program designed to provide the family physician in training with an outpatient clinical experience as part of a nequipo team in the treatment of couples in short-term group psychotherapy.* The unique educational experience allowed participating family practice residents to develop some familiarity with the range of presenting complaints often seen with troubled relationships and to develop comfort in approaching psychosocial issues with patients that they would be likely to treat in their practice of family medicine. Although proficiency as a psychotherapist was not a goal of the residents, awareness of both healthy and unhealthy dynamics in couple communication was a desired outcome.

In one case, Rob, a highly motivated and intelligent family practice resident, was selected by Leah, a knowledgeable and experienced psychotherapist who had created the program, to be her partner in a nequipo team. Leah was an outstanding teacher who understood the value of peer consultation. She invited Bill to act as their clinical guide in the area of shared group leadership. Bill was present as a consultant in the first couples' group they led, and once their nequipo relationship was developed, they conducted their second couples' group without his presence. Several obstacles had to be overcome in the successful functioning of the nequipo team. In the beginning, Leah tended to "de-skill" herself in a well-intended effort to make the nequipo team more balanced. She would delay timely interventions with the couples and defer their questions to Rob in an effort to include him in the group process.

During post-group sessions, Bill explored with Rob his apprehensions at being a novice in group. He helped him set aside the cumbersome expectation that he should act as an authority and, thereby, freed him to show more of himself. As Rob became more active and assertive as a person, Leah was relieved to discover that she could retain her skills as a clinician and not overshadow him as she had feared. She did know much more than he in the area of family dynamics and possessed superior clinical acumen, and neither she nor Rob gained by concealing the fact.

Another obstacle was the couples' tendency to direct their questions about medicine and medical treatment to Rob once they learned he was

*A detailed account of this innovative program is given by Ruben Contreras, MD, MPH and Lee Scheingold, MSW, in their article, "Couples Groups in Family Practice Training," *The Journal of Family Practice*, Vol. 18, No. 2:293–296, 1984.

a physician. This became a tricky problem for the nequipos to solve, since Rob's initial credibility in group was based on his medical credentials. If he indulged the patients' questions, which in terms of group process amounted to supporting their avoidance of psychological topics, he undermined the purpose of the group. If he declined to answer them, he felt uncomfortable withholding information in his area of expertise. The nequipos developed a creative solution to this dilemma by reframing the patients' questions to include the psychosocial context. For example, the question, "What medications would help me sleep at night?" became "What stresses in my family and relationship are keeping me awake?" Rob emphasized that he was in the group to learn about couples and that he needed to listen to *them* in order to achieve his goal.

### Co-Therapists Who Became Nequipos and Vice-Versa

Vivian participated in two divergent nequipo teams during a 2-year period. The first team, Vivian and Brad, was meant to be a bona fide co-therapy relationship but turned into a nequipo failure. The second team, Vivian and Melissa, was intended to be a standard nequipo arrangement but turned into a sparkling collaborative success when Melissa approached Vivian's level of ability much more quickly than anticipated.

In the first case, Vivian chose Brad to conduct a group with her in full expectation that he would be her equal. They had both practiced as licensed therapists for an equal number of years, and they both had similar academic credentials. Both had practiced group therapy for several years. Although Vivian had 5 years of co-leadership experience and Brad had less than a year, she assumed he would catch up speedily. In addition, Vivian thought he would bring a welcome dose of humor and lightness to the emotionally intense group that she put together and led herself. She perceived Brad to be ambitious and eager to be financially successful.

The enterprise started well, and Brad made his initial connections to group members gracefully. However, problems began to emerge as the group went deeper into its process. As the unconscious conflicts unfolded, Brad became progressively withdrawn. At first his passivity was interpreted by Vivian as a calculated observational stance. However, as his silence persisted, Vivian began to question him in post-group sessions. It became clear that Brad's therapeutic style was radically different from his personal style. Although pleasant and warm socially, he became frozen in session. After 6 months of frustrating co-leadership, Brad suggested that he attempt to balance the power in the team by taking on maintenance functions such as starting and stopping the group and keeping the books. Vivian greeted these attempts optimistically but soon discovered they were merely cosmetic alterations. When Vivian was away on vacation a conflict ensued between two clients that Brad did not handle well. On her return, Vivian attempted to mend the breach but found it was too late. The group dissolved, and with it the imbalanced co-therapy relationship.

In the second case, Vivian selected an intern under her supervision whose work she had closely observed and admired. Vivian wanted to co-lead a women's group with Melissa as her nequipo because she demonstrated the qualities that Vivian desired in a co-therapist: intuitive abilities, willingness to nurture, and patience that did not preclude being active. Two months into the group she began to receive dividends she had not expected. Melissa brought referrals into the group. She brought enthusiasm and equal energy. By following Melissa's lead, Vivian further developed her own intuition. By the end of the first year, Melissa seemed less like a nequipo and more like a co-therapist. After Melissa became licensed, they became bona fide co-therapists with a growing friendship.

The case of Brad illustrates that knowing someone personally is not a sufficient reason to select him or her as a co-therapist. One must know his or her style and behavior as a clinician. Vivian had this information about Melissa when she chose her as a nequipo, and the results were propitious.

### Training a Member of the Support Staff

Bill invited Adrianne to join him as an assistant therapist in a group designed especially for depressed women facing crises in their lives. Adrianne was an untrained but highly talented member of the support staff of a large mental health service that treated patients drawn from a large metropolitan area. Her job was answering phone calls and scheduling appointments with appropriate clinicians based on the information she obtained in her phone interviews. She had demonstrated considerable ability dealing with individuals in crisis, and she possessed accurate although informal diagnostic skills based on her acute intuitive sense of people. Bill selected her as his assistant because she was motivated to learn and willing to make a commitment of 1 year as his protege. He knew that Adrianne would be the first to make contact with most new members by way of their crisis calls to her. Her presence in the group would provide a welcome sense of continuity with the voice patients had first heard on the phone.

The group proved quite demanding and soon put the skills of both leaders to the test. In the second month of the group's operation, it was discovered through a series of personal breakthroughs and revelations that every woman in the group had been sexually abused as a child. Some had known this prior to entry in the group, but others had uncovered the fact of abuse when the influence of the group helped rupture their walls of denial. Adrianne had grasped the nature of the group intuitively before the fact became known to the group, and she assisted in the powerful transformation that occurred in the group's structure. She helped the group perceive Bill as a kind and nurturing male, a task that would have been quite impossible for Bill to have done on his own, given the stark history of the women in the group. In supervision, Bill helped Adrianne establish her boundaries as a leader in the group, since she had a tendency to identify too strongly with the women. He interpreted her strong countertransference reactions and dreams so that she increased her professional distance. Both leaders helped each other track the many projections hurled at them by anxious and suffering group members.

Over the course of a year, the ego strength of the patients increased, and they made healthy behavioral changes in their lives. In one woman, the breakthrough to unconscious material was so painful that she attempted suicide. She had called Adrianne at home early Sunday morning, a little past midnight just before ingesting barbiturates. Adrianne awakened Bill with a call, and together they entered the patient's home to bring emergency medical assistance. In this way, the nequipo unit functioned effectively as a crisis team, although typically not in such a dramatic fashion.


## CO-LEARNER TEAMS IN ACTION

Co-learner teams are also common in training settings and present many challenges to the co-learners and their supervisors. Below are vignettes of co-learners at work. The first continues the narrative immediately above.

### A Nequipo Who Became a Co-Learner

When Adrianne's year commitment had come to an end, she wanted to return to school and study psychology. She also wanted to continue with the group. Bill needed to leave the group to begin another within the service. He recognized the special purpose of the group within the mental health system and knew that it should continue as a service to consumers. He chose Sheila to replace him as Adrianne's partner in the group and became the supervisor of the newly formed co-learner team. This co-learner team did not have equal status at the beginning of their supervision because Adrianne, although still very much a student, had become more of a friend and colleague of Bill's during their intense work together. This situation presented a challenge to Sheila, who did not have a history with the women's group and, because she was new to the service, had not had the opportunity of a nequipo relationship with Bill. Bill chose Sheila to co-lead the group because she was completing her Master's degree in psychology and had experience in crisis intervention. Along with her personal qualities of maturity and confidence, she brought many gifts to the co-learner relationship that compensated for her newness in the group. Bill believed she was powerful enough to create a balanced co-learner team.

Bill faced a challenge, too. He had to set more distant boundaries on his personal relationship with Adrianne in order to establish his role as supervisor. During supervisory sessions, he intentionally became more silent and removed while Adrianne and Sheila discussed the group. Adrianne would ask Bill questions about the group, and instead of responding, he would invite Sheila to share her perceptions with Adrianne. This was done in order to interrupt the ease and familiarity of the nequipo arrangement and allow Sheila to develop a co-learner relationship with Adrianne. By these means, Bill attempted to treat both co-learners equally during supervision and avoided conferring special status to Adrianne because of their previous collaboration.

Gradually Sheila earned the respect of the group members as they came to admire her individuality and tough-mindedness. Sheila and Adrianne initiated a process in the women's group that went beyond the achievements of the nequipo team. Whereas the group had explored their relationship to the abusing males under the leadership of Bill and Adrianne, with Adrianne and Sheila, they began to expose the role of mothers in the abusive family. The co-learners had achieved equal status.

### Co-Learners Who Hide Their Troubles from Their Supervisor

This example involves our colleague Ed, who, in his capacity as a clinical professor of psychiatry at a medical center, supervised a male–female co-learner team, Pamela and Michael. Ed met with them each week in group supervision with other co-learners and also met with them each week as a dyad. Together they were leading a year-long treatment group. Michael was a senior psychiatric resident and highly respected by the faculty for his clinical acumen and intelligence. He appeared confident and self-assured in his presentation. Pamela was a PhD candidate in psychology who was recognized for her outstanding academic record and ability as a writer. She seemed a modest person who skillfully focused attention on her patients and did not draw attention to herself.

Following the sixth meeting of their treatment group, Pamela pointed out to Michael his tendency to control the group by taking attention away from the group's own process. Each time the group entered a thoughtful silence, he would break the mood with a comment. Much to her surprise he lashed back at her defensively, stating, "That's absurd! What's wrong with you?" Pamela backed off from further confrontation and allowed Michael to dominate the group. In subsequent supervisory sessions neither mentioned the altercation. Michael felt he had won and saw no need for further discussion. Pamela was afraid to raise the issue because she believed Ed would support Michael's view.

As supervision continued, Ed received no clue of the troubles that beset the co-learners even though both submitted separate process notes every week as required. They denied having any difficulties in their relationship in their discussions with Ed, and he detected no acrimony between them. As always, Michael talked more during supervision whereas Pamela confined her comments to astute observations concerning the patients.

At the end of the training year, when the treatment groups had been terminated and all supervision was completed and the various co-learner teams disbanded, Ed learned the truth. By chance he met Pamela on the campus and complimented her for her final summary of the group. At the compliment, she burst into tears, protesting that it was all a sham. She proceeded to confess how unhappy she had been as a co-learner with Michael and related the events just described. Ed was astonished by her revelation and, as he listened, began to piece together how his supervision had gone awry. It occurred to him that co-learners may be too conflicted to share their difficulties with their supervisor in the presence of their partner. He soberly discovered and passed along the wisdom that individual sessions with each co-learner on an intermittent basis were a necessary part of the supervisory process, so each has an opportunity to break through denial.

### Countertransference

Julie and Sally had formed a co-learner team in the treatment of several families during their first year as interns at the student mental health service attached to the university. They were both in their early 20s, bright and highly motivated to learn. In the second year of their postgraduate training, they approached Bill to supervise them as co-learners in a group they wanted to start for undergraduate women at the university who suffered from a variety of anxiety disorders, including agoraphobia. Many of the women they accepted into their group also experienced quite a bit of difficulty forming relationships with men.

Bill found them a delighful co-learner team to supervise. He could see that they had advanced rapidly in their working relationship during their first year together, and he anticipated that they would progress even more as leaders of the women's group. In the early phases of the group, the women focused on the themes of career and their relationships with parents. The group soon discovered that most members came from alcoholic families of origin. This became an important topic for supervision, since both Julie and Sally had alcoholic fathers. They seemed to manage their boundaries very well in group and usually were able to monitor their own projections as a team onto members of the group. However, when the theme of the group switched to relationships with boyfriends, the co-learners' boundaries loosened.

Julie came to a supervisory session furious at Anabelle, one of the patients in the group, who had dropped two classes at the university in order to work more and support her lover who was a full-time student. "How could she do that?" fumed Julie. Sally was angry also, but with another client, Cal, who gave some of her weekly earnings to support her boyfriend's taste for expensive drugs. Both co-learners were livid and had not concealed in group their personal disapproval of the two women's actions. Bill asked probing questions about how the group members' behavior had brought up memories in the co-learners, but his queries were met by their blank, unfeeling stares. In subsequent sessions, both Sally and Julie reported that the group "seemed to be distancing" from the leaders. When Bill suggested this might be the co-learners' projection onto the group, they expressed a feeling that he was judging them negatively and that he did not appreciate their skill as co-leaders.

Bill interpreted the transference and suggested that each was placing her father's critical visage onto him. Julie admitted that it might be true and then added, ". . . and Anabelle reminds me of my mother, always sacrificing for Dad." Sally confessed a similar countertransferential reaction to Cal and marveled that she had not seen it before. This was a blind spot for both co-learners that they had not detected in each other, let alone themselves. Once it was identified, they were able to reinforce their boundaries with the group and become effective leaders once more.

### Competition with the Supervisor

Bill supervised a co-learner team composed of Bret and Frank, both older males and former athletes who possessed strong competitive urges. The co-learners chose each other because they liked each other, and they wanted to lead a year-long group for 13- and 14-year-old boys. They believed they could become positive role models for the boys, most of whom had no fathers at home.

Bill believed these men could work together because they had shared similar life experiences and seemed to agree on ways to set limits on acting out by adolescents.

During the first supervisory session the co-learners presented such divergent pictures of the group process that Bill could not ascertain what actually had happened. Both co-learners exhibited a stubborn unwillingness to shift their points of view in order to clarify the events that had occurred. At Bill's suggestion, they began videotaping sessions for discussion in supervision. The tapes helped Bill, but they did not seem to affect the co-learners' inability to agree. They independently developed creative methods to stem acting out in the group but were unable to settle on a single plan of action. Bret suggested using batakas, or foam rubber bats, to allow the boys to fight each other and drain off excess adolescent energy. Frank wanted the boys to play basketball as a way to express their aggression. Bill convinced them that the activities were not mutually exclusive and encouraged them to proceed.

The boys liked the activities and, following them, appeared more available emotionally to discuss their problems. However, the co-learners were not available to the boys because they had become so engrossed in the activities that they competed between themselves like two Dads coaching soccer. Bill confronted the co-learners and told them they were using their patients to express their competitive tendencies. Both co-learners turned on Bill and told him he was wrong. They were teaching the boys healthy expressions of aggression, and they implied that they knew more about that than Bill. Bill responded to their competitive challenge inappropriately by becoming competitive himself. Rather than returning the focus of the therapy to the needs of the adolescents, he entered the competition for who could provide the best model for being a male. Whereas the original purpose of the therapy was to help the boys control their impulses, the supervisory sessions became centered on which male could best teach the boys control.

During one supervisory session, Bill challenged both co-learners to a game of ping-pong. In the middle of a hard-fought game, he realized the supervision had gone off track, and he was engaging in adolescent acting out himself. He said this to Frank and Bret, and they both laughed a laugh of recognition. The task of supervision became clear. It was Bill's job to help the co-learners become a cooperative team so that they could assist the boys to work cooperatively in group.

### Competition for the Praise of the Supervisor

Many years ago, when Vivian was in graduate school, she and Anita became co-learners in the treatment of a family and participated together in once-a-week supervision with Wilfred, a well-established family therapist. Both Vivian and Anita showed much enthusiasm for family therapy and enjoyed the opportunity to learn from Wilfred. During individual supervision, Vivian felt competent and acknowledged by Wilfred. However, in conjoint supervision with Anita, Vivian became unsure of herself and her abilities. Anita brought to each supervisory session a creative exercise for the family to implement that week. She bestowed these exercises on Wilfred as gifts a loving daughter might offer her father. Vivian saw Wilfred's delight in Anita's contributions and attempted to invent exercises in order to please him. However, in Vivian's eyes her efforts never appeared to match Anita's brilliance. In fact, Vivian's forte was developing insights about the family system based on her ability to analyze. In her competition with Anita she lost sight of her own proficiency.

Wilfred appeared to relish the attention showed him by both women. He did not seem aware of the competition between them for his approval and did not interpret the transference that lay at its heart. In the beginning Vivian and Anita had liked each other, but tension between them began to show in the treatment of the family. They did not interact as much in sessions, nor did they model cooperativeness of spirit. The co-learners' attention was on themselves and their supervisor, and not on the concerns of the family in treatment. In the interest of the family therapy, the co-learners struck on a new agreement whereby Vivian would use Anita's exercises and Anita would honor Vivian's interpretations. They, in effect, discovered a strategy of complementarity in order to serve the family better. Like loyal daughters, they never bothered Wilfred with this problem, and so he remained ideal in their imaginations. Wilfred never inquired about the relationship between the co-learners, but fortunately they came to a resolution on their own. A year later Vivian repeated the same issue with another supervisor who pointed out her transference, and she sought psychotherapy to address the unresolved archaic material between father and daughter.

## Supervisor's Countertransference

Sandy and Nell were co-learners in the treatment of a family whose identified patient was a 14-year-old girl named Gina. Her mother claimed that Gina was "incorrigible" and "uncontrollable" because she stayed out all night and refused to follow the rules of the family. Mother was particularly upset that Gina was associating with "strange men" twice her age and had admitted to being sexual with some of them. Gina had two younger sisters, and Mother was afraid that they would follow her example. In the first family session, the father alternated between being angry at Gina "for disrupting the family peace" and passively withdrawing after the statement "She's a rotten apple just like my sister."

In supervision, the co-learners were advised to explore the father's family of origin, especially his relationship with his mother. In subsequent sessions, Raymond, their supervisor and director of the family therapy program, spent a considerable amount of time analyzing the behavior of the father. When Nell pointed out that Gina seemed to be lost in their discussion of the family, he responded defensively that if she wanted to learn about family therapy, she should listen to him. Following his directions, the co-learners focused their energy on increasing the father's authority in the family in order to balance his wife's tendency to take control. This strategy had positive results for the couple, but Gina's acting out only escalated.

Sandy and Nell discussed the case together and decided to confront Raymond about his neglect of Gina. Again Raymond responded defensively, discounting the ideas of the two co-learners as adolescent acting out. He believed they were questioning his authority as a way to build an alliance for themselves and avoid a deeper analysis of their working relationship as co-learners. The co-learners were not dissuaded, and they stood their ground. Sandy stated, "This isn't about us, this is about a daughter wanting to be closer to her father and a father not letting her. I can identify with Gina and feel her frustration."

As Sandy spoke, Raymond was startled by how similar her words were to those of his wife, who only yesterday entreated him to acknowledge the burgeoning womanhood of their own 14-year-old daughter. He reflected on how much his distant relationship with their daughter was troubling him. He candidly replied to Nell, "Perhaps I am projecting my own experience onto the family." Together with the co-learners, Raymond began to reconsider the needs of Gina in the context of the family. The co-learners implemented timely and appropriate interventions, and the relationship between Gina and her father began to improve. Within the family's new structure, her compulsion to act out was greatly diminished.

Raymond acknowledged the contribution of the co-learners to the family's progress. Their assertiveness had helped him to see his own countertransference. Sandy had learned to trust her empathy because it had led to the uncovering of the countertransference. Both benefited from Raymond's modeling of openness and his ability to scrutinize his own personal involvement in the case. He had acted in exemplary fashion by listening to the co-learners and respecting their views.

### Co-Dependency between Co-Learners

Molly and Saul were co-learners employed as part of the staff of a major mental health institute and were students in its family therapy training program. They had chosen to work together and were assigned to a couple whose 4-year-old child had died 2 years before. The couple had received crisis counseling throughout the child's prolonged illness and grief counseling after his death. Despite a considerable amount of therapy, the couple remained troubled. They had a history of fighting with their therapists and devaluing their efforts to help them. Molly and Saul had been chosen to work with this family by their supervisor, Anastasia, because she believed they were highly advanced students and could handle a challenge of this magnitude.

In the first session, the father and mother recounted the history of how several therapists had failed to help them. They maintained that the death of little Joey was no longer a problem for them, although the very mention of Joey set them off into a tirade against the doctors and the medical establishment. They said their problem was that they were not able to become pregnant, and for that reason, they fought a good deal. It appeared to the co-learners that the only emotional connection that they shared was their animosity toward physicians. They did not touch each other or make eye contact but rather addressed their comments to the co-learners as if they expected a decision from them about who was right.

In supervision Anastasia asked the co-learners how they were going to begin questioning the assumptions of their couple. Both Saul and Molly said they preferred to move slowly in that area. They both expressed fear that if they confronted too soon, the couple would direct their anger at them. They wanted to proceed with caution and keep the couple from fleeing therapy. As the weeks went by, they took no steps toward challenging their clients' misperceptions. When Anastasia asked them how they planned to break the impasse, the co-learners looked at each other with apprehension. It became clear to Anastasia that they were colluding to support each other's overly cautious stance. Anastasia showed how they were being manipulated by the couple's anger and how the anger served to perpetuate the family's suffering. "You must help the parents challenge the belief that they can keep their child alive by staying angry."

Although they found Anastasia's argument intellectually compelling, the co-learners resisted taking risks in the service of advancing the therapy. The co-learners had become as co-dependent in their own way as the couple in treatment with them. Anastasia began to treat the co-learner team for their co-dependency. In this way she modeled how to approach the co-dependent couple. She instructed the co-learners to look at their similarities and differences as people. They realized that part of the reason they had chosen each other as co-learners was their tendency to avoid risks. Neither saw himself or herself as courageous, and they did not encourage each other to move into areas where they might fail as former therapists had. Anastasia asked them to look at the consequences of what they called "failure." What emerged for them were images of parental disapproval. Both had felt it was better to remain frozen than face parental disappointment. Fortunately, Anastasia was willing to be a parental figure who approved responsible risk taking and shared with them some of her own mistakes and how she had learned by them.

Saul and Molly responded positively by returning to the couple and asking them if they believed they had failed Joey and each other by his death. This intervention opened a new realm for discussion and led to the expression of sadness and to a deep introspection by the couple on how they had failed. This initial success inspired the co-learners to become more therapeutically assertive, which produced positive results. For the first time the couple showed empathy for each other's grief by touching hands gently and making tender eye contact. Once the couple could move beyond their anger at others and their denial of Joey's death, they could begin to mourn their lost child and lovingly approach the creation of another.

# • 3 •

# *How to Choose a Co-Therapist*

Our survey produced no evidence that co-therapy is the treatment of choice for any particular mental disorder or set of patients. And yet our respondents gave ample testimony for why therapists continue to choose co-therapy practice. Once co-therapy is chosen as a treatment strategy, co-therapists must choose each other.

We found that nearly two thirds of our survey sample chose the person or persons with whom they conducted co-therapy rather than being assigned (see Appendix). We expected this, since two thirds of our sample were in private practice and in a position to choose with whom they worked more often than therapists in institutional practice. This factor was a significant demographic characteristic of our sample and distinguished it from much previous research in the field in which therapists were assigned to their dyads.

It also became clear from our sample that experienced co-therapists know precisely what they want in a co-therapist. If given the choice, therapists will determine for themselves what they need in a professional partner. Assignment to a partner diminishes the autonomy experienced by the therapist and reduces the likelihood of a harmonious match. In this case, we believe there is less investment by each therapist in the outcome of their collaboration. They do not feel equally responsible for the pairing that has been created, and their commitment to the resolution of differences for the sake of the treatment process is not substantial. In some cases, the only thing they may jointly agree on is getting the experience over with as soon as possible.

For these reasons and others specified below, we believe that to choose one's co-therapist is a strongly preferred option. Furthermore, we believe that one's choice has clinical implications for the fate of the co-therapy and the therapy.

Co-therapy teams can be formed in three ways:

1. A solo therapist begins a course of individual, family or group therapy and invites a second therapist to join him or her.
2. Two therapists begin a course of therapy together.
3. An existing co-therapy team dissolves, and a new co-therapist joins the remaining therapist in on-going treatment of the same patients.

The replacement of one co-therapist by another is the most complex emotionally of the ways to begin co-therapy. The conditions that attend the dissolution of the co-therapy partnership, from the death of a co-therapist to the departure of the co-therapist to another geographic region, are critical and affect the new partnership and the clients who remain in treatment. The therapist must welcome his or her new partner and help the clients grieve the loss of the previous partner.

The death of a co-therapist is an agonizing experience for both patients and surviving co-therapist (Rosenthall, 1946). In contrast to a solo-led therapy group that must face the death of their therapist alone, the co-led group has the assistance of the co-therapist in their process of bereavement. The surviving therapist must select a person who can withstand the anger of the clients and empathize with their sadness. This person must bear up under frequent comparison to the lost and often idealized leader. He or she must project a strong personality and sense of self-esteem. The surviving therapist chooses a co-therapist not to replace the old team but to found a new one.

## QUALITIES THAT THERAPISTS DESIRE IN CO-THERAPISTS

The quality most frequently mentioned by the respondents to our survey was the capacity to be equal in communicating and openness. This was further elaborated as the ability to be comfortable asking questions of his or her partner in order to critique his or her attributes. The willingness to disagree or agree with a co-therapist outside the therapy session when differences emerge was thought to be important. Openness to the discussion of theoretical and interpersonal issues contributed to the constructive management of differences. They expected a co-therapist to confront them as well as to provide support. Of particular value was an openness to discuss the co-therapy relationship. They also desired someone willing to share treatment objectives and develop common goals. Some group therapists in particular wanted co-therapists who would disclose themselves in a group and be an authentic person and not a blank screen. Co-therapists wanted a person who could process with them after a treatment session and formulate a sense of what happened. The capacity to differ openly was valued, and the ability to confront with empathy was highly esteemed. These observations are consonant with our own encounters with many co-therapists.

The qualities of being equal in power, noncompetitive (relatively), and compatible also received many votes. Co-therapists wanted especially to avoid power struggles because these cancel out the effectiveness of the treatment process and drain the energy of the co-therapists. Whereas a totally noncompetitive pairing was neither possible nor necessarily desirable, a relative absence of rivalrous feelings was thought to be obtainable. Some similarity in style of practice and technique was judged good. But the ability to mesh therapeutic efforts whatever one's approach was clearly favored. The highly subjective notion of a "compatible personality" was deemed important. This meant a person who was both intellectually and emotionally compatible. An overall commitment to teamwork and cooperation is desirable.

Co-therapists preferred professionals who possess a number of discrete skills. They favored someone with a "depth of experience." They also mentioned similar levels of experience as desirable, but we have found that a similar level of experience is not necessary in a co-therapist. Much more significant is the capacity to grasp profound moments in therapy and understand their significance for the course of the treatment. Professionals want partners who possess professional attitudes. These attitudes include taking responsibility for the course and progress of treatment and taking corrective action when necessary. These attitudes define what is considered competence and are demonstrated by a person's maturity in carrying out therapeutic interventions. Together these concepts constitute what is meant by being "well trained," and we see them clearly or note their absence when we work with a co-therapist.

Co-therapists prefer a similar theoretical orientation in their partners and, to some degree, a similar set of values as persons. Comments by our respondents ranged from one person who expected the same theoretical viewpoint in a partner to another who wanted a co-therapist with a similar philosophy of life. Many look for a similar sense of values and define that as a harmony of ideas about how people change and how the human condition is perceived. Group therapists particularly wanted a co-therapist in tune with their own theories about group therapy. Respondents believed it would be easier to share authority with a person with whom they share basic assumptions. In particular, they believed that similar basic assumptions would allow them to formulate therapeutic goals and develop treatment plans.

Two other personal traits most often sought were empathy and sensitivity. These were thought to be especially helpful in the treatment of patients as well as important in working through conflicts in the co-therapy relationship. Therapists wanted co-therapists who were able to sense the feelings of their patients and be attuned to the feelings of their partners. A general awareness of the feeling component was given strong approval.

It is pertinent to note that three of the five categories of desirable traits are abilities that any therapist must bring to the task of psychotherapy. Only the choices of equality in communication and equality of power relate specifically to the task of co-therapy because they require the context of a relationship to be implemented. It is of interest to us that therapists expect more of the professionals they choose as their co-therapists than they want of professionals to whom they refer patients. They do not demand these extra abilities from the latter group.

## QUALITIES THAT THERAPISTS BRING TO CO-THERAPY

Our sample demonstrated their considerable tenure as working professionals by indicating that experience in therapy, co-therapy, and group therapy was the chief asset they brought to the co-therapy team. Interestingly, experience did not appear as a highly desired trait from their point of view, but it was clearly what they believed they had to offer. Co-therapists must bring gifts to the co-therapy setting, but in some cases it appears that the gift a person brings may not be the gift most desired. This demonstrates the need for potential co-therapists to discuss their desires and assets at the start of the relationship in order to address expectations and assumptions on the part of both. We expand on this notion in our discussion of the uses of the Co-Therapy Issues Questionnaire later in this chapter.

Respondents did indicate that skills were an important asset that they provided, just as skills were also a desirable commodity in their partners. Their skills included both clinical acumen and counseling abilities.

Knowledge of group therapy and knowledge as a professional with a breadth of training were also cited. Respondents believed that much of their knowledge was based on clinical experience. The statement "I know things my co-therapist doesn't" was typical.

Respondents also listed a capacity to work cooperatively as a major asset. They believed this was manifest in their cooperative attitude and relative absence of rivalrous feelings. They were able to foster a spirit of collaboration and be an effective team member. Teamwork is the key idea, and these therapists contribute to its development.

Although our sample listed open communication as the most desired quality in a co-therapist, most respondents did not place that quality nearly as high in the list of what they had to give. In this manner, we perceive how therapists attempt to balance their abilities in their selection of a co-therapist. This demonstrates the principle of balancing which is a chief element in the success of a co-therapy team as we discuss in Chapter 4. Those people who believed they could provide open communication defined it as the ability to request and accept feedback and the ability to give and take direction from their co-therapist as needed. Open communication also implied the willingness to negotiate differences, to examine oneself, and to work out interpersonal dynamics with a co-leader. Respondents also said they could admit mistakes and believed that doing so contributed significantly to a good co-therapy relationship. They were willing to initiate discussion with their co-therapists and confront them with empathy when they differed in beliefs or operating procedures.

Responding therapists indicated their willingness to acknowledge differences and to learn new approaches to therapy. Their flexibility was manifest in a willingness to adapt co-therapy treatment to various modes of psychotherapy. As part of a co-therapy team, they were willing to experiment with new techniques and to some degree change their own style of practice. They did this not only to suit a new partner but also to relax their own professional rigidity. By these means, we see them reaffirming their chief reason for choosing co-therapy practice: to learn from their co-therapist.

As experienced practitioners in the field, our therapists stated they could be comfortable with themselves, and their feeling of comfort was based on their confidence and self-esteem. In several examples, women stated they were comfortable as strong females modeling for other women. Their sense of personal and professional accomplishment was well established within themselves and manifested in their personal integrity. Good psychological boundaries and a well-developed sense of personal security were both assets they brought to co-therapy.

Interestingly, some therapists spoke not only of believing themselves competent but also of being competent with their feelings. In other words, their ability to be cognizant of their own feelings and their ability to accept themselves and their feelings were two defining characteristics of their competence.

The capacity to be sensitive to patients, to oneself, and to one's co-therapist was mentioned. Sensitivity had also been chosen as a trait desired in a co-therapist. Yet, it is curious that with an older, mature sample, experience is clearly given greater value than sensitivity. In that regard, we are left with the impression that people may enter the field of psychotherapy with sensitivity but leave with experience. Whether true or not, this is a striking exchange of attitudes that may occur during the course of professional life and is a fascinating notion on which to speculate. It is possible that the theoretical orientation of our sample influences this outcome. This is a variable that lies outside the scope of our study but warrants further investigation.

Responding therapists also indicated a willingness to share gifts with their co-therapists. Specifically, the gifts shared were observations, feedback, and new information. But generally, they meant sharing a certain generosity of spirit that pervaded their interactions with a co-therapist. This factor, we believe, elevates the level at which the co-therapy team is functioning and is clearly seen by patients and colleagues who have an opportunity to view their interactions.

We find it interesting to note that six of the nine categories of gifts co-therapists bring to their team are qualities they must bring to the task of psychotherapy and are not related specifically to the practice of co-therapy. What are specific to co-therapy are the capacity to work cooperatively, open communication, and willingness to share gifts. These qualities require a relationship with another therapist to put into effect. They are critical factors in co-therapy and require energy and attention on the part of the practitioner. A psychotherapist expects more of him- or herself in the role of co-therapist than in solo practice. This may in part account for some therapists choosing not to practice co-therapy. A self-selective process is probably at work. Those who want to make these critical factors a part of their work life will seek out co-therapy as an opportunity to have them fulfilled.

When our respondents referred to their desire for open communication with a partner and their capacity to supply it themselves, their comments reflected a stunning similarity. In selecting co-therapists, therapists look for some of the traits that they themselves offer. But there is a more significant point. In psychotherapy, each therapist can bring different qualities to his or her clients and still prove successful.

Yet, in co-therapy, therapists must bring a critical number of similar qualities to the relationship if that relationship is to be successful. We speak more of this principle and supply examples in Chapter 4.

There are many other assets that clinicians can bring to the co-therapy dyad. Possessing an outgoing personality and the capacity simply to take pleasure in the person of one's co-therapist are assets. The ability to mesh therapeutic efforts and strike a good balance is another. Respect for one's co-therapist was interpreted as an asset. And yet this respect was not blind to faults. A sharp awareness of liabilities in a partner as well as his or her assets was considered desirable.


## SEX AS A CRITERION FOR CHOICE

In our study, striking a sexual balance was deemed important. Only two people, one man and one woman, preferred a same-sex co-therapist. This was clearly an idiosyncratic response for our sample, although it was not statistically significant (see Appendix). The majority of our therapists responding to this question preferred the opposite sex in their co-therapist choices as shown in the summary below.

Preferred sex of co-therapist

| | |
|---|---|
| The number preferring opposite sex: | 26 men and 21 women |
| The number preferring same sex: | 1 man and 1 woman |
| The number expressing equal preference between the sexes: | 20 men and 9 women |
| TOTAL | 47 men and 31 women |

It is noteworthy that women were more likely to choose an opposite-sex co-therapist than men. Among the 31 women, opposite-sex co-therapy teams were preferred two to one. Although this result was not statistically significant (see Appendix), it is still tempting to speculate on this outcome. Why did males choose women less frequently for partners than women chose men?

One interpretation of this phenomenon is the notion of "male superiority." This interpretation would favor the notion that males have greater respect for other males' abilities, and their choice is an expression of that respect. Presumably, women also respect the males' abilities, perhaps more so than those of their own sex. We believe that this interpetation of data is highly improbable in view of this sample's expressed interest in the notion of equality as a condition for the practice of co-therapy. It is entirely possible that some of our sample, both male and female, do not view male and female therapists as equals. But we do not think that sexual prejudice is surfacing in the way people responded to this particular question. There are factors other than belief in equality or inequality that produce this outcome.

A closer study of the comments showed that both male and female therapists cared equally for the notion of striking a sexual balance in the team and for the idea of stimulating parental transference. But seven women named modeling male–female communication as a criterion whereas only two men did so. The women cited "model of family," "model as parent figures and as a couple," and "better modeling of complementarity" as their reasons. The two male therapists simply stated "two sex models" were desirable. How do we interpret this?

We can assume that most people in our society had many female figures, either caretakers or teachers, in the pre-oedipal and oedipal phases of childhood development and one or no male models. Perhaps in light of the relative absence of males in the rearing of children and during their early education, women therapists may say, "Our patients, both men and women, need males in their psychological lives, and we shall provide them with it." Satir's comments in Chapter 9 of this volume point to this need in our society and support this interpretation of the data. In the transference phenomenon, either sex will do as the object of transference. But for modeling sex-linked behavior, the patient must have a specific representative of the sex. Presumably, therapists of both sexes consider modeling important, but male therapists are able to fill this absence, whereas female therapists must seek out the male presence for their patients.

Of those therapists with equal preference between sexes, most stated it simply "did not make a difference" to them. Many said it depended on the situation of the clients they were treating. For example, one therapist reported, "couples sometimes feel more represented with a female and a male," whereas "female incest groups are more comfortable with two women therapists." However, no consensus was detected in our sample on the appropriateness of same-sex/opposite-sex teams for specific treatment conditions or patients.

## PRACTICAL INSTRUMENTS AND EXERCISES FOR SELECTING A CO-THERAPIST

For 12 years we have employed two exercises and a questionnaire of co-therapy issues to stimulate discussion on the choice of a co-therapist. These procedures were first used to bring to the surface some of the many topics that co-therapists must talk about if they are going to negotiate a co-therapy contract and initiate a working co-therapy relationship. With some adaptations, the questionnaire and exercises can be utilized in the formation of both nequipo (not equal) and co-learner (non-therapist) teams. We have also found that these procedures can help existing co-therapy relationships by focusing attention on issues unconsciously avoided or neglected by the distraction of everyday work schedules. Again, therapists must remember: the co-therapy relationship will never take care of itself; it must be given attention, especially at the beginning.

How do we apply the questionnaire and use the exercises? In training and consulting with co-therapists, we give the Co-Therapy Issues Questionnaire to prospective co-therapy candidates to be completed by them before meeting together to discuss responses. Each person records his or her responses to each question and then confers with his or her partner-to-be. The most obvious use of the questionnaire is to compare positive and negative responses. But the really helpful process is the dialogue that ensues. In this dialogue, each person can explore various aspects of the other's personality and professional preferences. Shades of meaning not possible to communicate in the questionnaire, become exposed. Soon the questionnaire can be set aside as the Zen teacher speaks of a *Koan*, simply as a brick to knock at a gate, and after the gate is opened to be discarded.

Creative co-therapists can and will develop their own means of opening the gates for communication. The questionnaire we offer here is one example of how two people can begin the process. Both nequipo and co-learner teams will also benefit from using the questionnaire.

## CO-THERAPY ISSUES QUESTIONNAIRE

In answering the following questions, you may find yourself in doubt over some. If you spend more than 50% of your time in an activity, answer "yes"; if you spend less than 50% of your time in an activity, answer "no". Likewise, if a question is more than 50% true for you, answer "yes"; if a question is less than 50% true for you, answer "no".

Record your co-therapist's or potential co-therapist's responses later, after he or she has completed the questionnaire separately.

In your work doing therapy:

1. Do you reveal yourself to patients (clients)?_____

               Co-therapist response_____

2. Are you adept at being empathic?_____

               Co-therapist response_____

3. Are you adept at being analytic?_____

    Co-therapist response_____

4. Do you use your imagination and fantasy in work?

    Co-therapist response_____

5. Are you confrontive in general?_____

    Co-therapist response_____

6. Are you supportive in general?_____

    Co-therapist response_____

7. Do you incline toward here-and-now interventions?_____

    Co-therapist response_____

8. Do you favor careful historical analysis of patient's life?_____

    Co-therapist response_____

9. Do you use religious beliefs as an approach to your client's life?_____

    Co-therapist response_____

10. Are you attuned to "psychic" phenomena with your patients?_____

    Co-therapist response_____

11. Do you believe divorce is a moral issue?_____

    Co-therapist response_____

12. Can you accept both traditional and nontraditional relationships between men and women?_____

    Co-therapist response_____

13. Are you willing to have a sliding scale in view of a client's ability to pay?_

14. Are you generally accepting of the people you see in therapy?_____

    Co-therapist response_____

15. Are you quietly enraged by a patient who lies and denies in the therapy session?_____

    Co-therapist response_____

16. Are you angered by silent and withdrawn clients?_____

    Co-therapist response_____

17. Do you prefer long-term or short-term therapy?_____

    Co-therapist response_____

18. Do you like to discuss theories and ideas about psychotherapy?_____

    Co-therapist response_____

19. Would you rather be doing some other kind of work than psycho-therapy?_____

Co-therapist response_____

20. Do you believe dreams are important in working through the conflicts of your patients?_____

Co-therapist response_____

21. Do you prefer group therapy to individual therapy as a form of treatment?_____

Co-therapist response_____

22. Do you feel competent as a family therapist?_____

Co-therapist response_____

Once the questionnaire has been discussed, we initiate two exercises with co-therapists. They assume a face-to-face sitting position, make eye contact, and talk directly to each other. The first exercise involves what each person wants in a co-therapist. Each person states this directly while his partner listens carefully but gives no feedback at that time. A reasonable time for each person to express his or her wants is five minutes. An opportunity to ask questions and clarify points is given immediately following the exercise. The initial purpose is to give and receive information. To say that you want something from your co-therapist does not imply a criticism. You may in fact want something that he or she is currently providing. A statement about wants is a statement about one's self and not a judgment of the other. A co-therapist cannot be faulted for failure to do something he or she did not know about. This exercise is very useful for first-time co-therapists, and it remains a powerful exercise for co-therapists to repeat with one another over time. What co-therapists want from each other can and does change over time with the growth of their relationship.

The second exercise is completed in the same manner as the first, with both therapists facing each other with eye contact. Only this time, the co-therapists will share what they are able and willing to provide in the co-therapy relationship. Again, five minutes should be devoted to each person separately to speak of his or her gifts while the partner listens carefully. The information that emerges from these exercises is most valuable and becomes the content for the contract that co-therapists negotiate for themselves.

## THE CO-THERAPY CONTRACT

We recommend that each co-therapy pair draw up a contract as a basis for the pair's work together. A contract allows much safety and freedom for the individuals within the relationship to grow. Such a contract can be more or less formal and more or less detailed, depending on the wishes of the co-therapists.

We suggest that the following points be considered by co-therapists as they negotiate the particulars of their contracts:

1. Both parties are equally responsible for monitoring the terms of this contract.
2. The parties shall enter into it as equal partners in every way unless otherwise specified.
3. The contract can be terminated at any time by either partner. Both parties agree that the association must be mutually rewarding, and if for any reason it is not, it can be ended. However, great consideration must be given to their clients for separation and closure if termination is agreed upon. Ideally, co-therapists should be discussing their dissatisfaction before termination becomes the issue.
4. If misunderstandings have developed, perhaps a new contract can be negotiated such that the co-therapy pairing may once again prove mutually beneficial.
5. Procedures for resolving differences and negotiating new contracts should be provided for. Third-party consulting, with a trusted colleague or associate, may prove helpful in this regard.
6. Frequent post-treatment discussions should be built into the operating procedures of the co-therapists. Mutual feedback and discussion of feelings should be incorporated as standard practice.
7. Both parties to the co-therapy agreement must share a similar idea of how co-therapy relationships can develop and a general idea of how they want their own relationship to develop. It is best to keep goals flexible, but it is also good to begin with some goals in terms of treatment plans and in terms of the co-therapy relationship.
8. Express congruence. Be frank about what you know and what you don't know.
9. Generously acknowledge your co-therapist for his or her contributions to your own learning.
10. Avoid unnecessary competition. The co-therapy relationship is fraught with opportunities to compete and upstage your partner. Most often, such acts will diminish the trust between co-therapists and produce resentment.
11. Establish psychological boundaries that are comfortable for both persons and permit a measure of intimacy that is mutually

acceptable to both and that does not compromise either individual's integrity or autonomy.

12. If co-therapists are associated for a year or more, significant time should be allotted to closure of the relationship and saying goodbye.

Once you have chosen both the practice of co-therapy and your co-therapist, some new questions emerge. What makes a particular co-therapy team successful? And what do we mean by success in the context of co-therapy? These are discussed in the chapter that follows.

# ◆ 4 ◆

# *Why a Co-Therapy Team Becomes Successful*

When we speak of the successful co-therapy team we mean the team that establishes a working contract, that matures in their work together over time, and that brings a modicum of benefit to their patients and a measure of satisfaction to themselves. What special conditions allow these felicitous events to occur?

As a starting point for our survey question concerning the factors of co-therapy success, we selected Herbert Rabin's excellent pioneer study of the attitudes of experienced group therapists (Rabin, 1967). We chose the six criteria that emerged from his study as most important in developing a co-therapy team in the context of a group and asked our respondents to rate them as factors that contributed to the success of the co-therapy team. This proved to be a wise choice, since our findings expanded on the useful conclusions of Rabin's study. Of particular interest was our corroboration of two factors that were clearly of little importance to overall success: the professional discipline of each co-therapist and the ages of the potential co-therapists.

The factors for success that emerged from our survey were as follows, in order of importance:

1. Complementary balance of therapist skills.
2. Compatibility of therapists' theoretical viewpoints.
3. Openness in communication.
4. Equality of participation.
5. Liking each other as people.
6. Respect.

Of these factors, numbers 1, 2, and 4 are present in Rabin's criteria, and we added numbers 3, 5, and 6 based on our respondents' thoughtful and detailed replies. Any working contract that co-therapists design for themselves should consider these factors. We shall demonstrate each success factor with examples from our own work as co-therapists.

## COMPLEMENTARY BALANCE OF SKILLS

Complementary balance of therapist skills was rated most important. This was a complex response and indicated the preference of our co-therapists for balance in how energy is expended and how an individual's actions complement his or her partner's.

We see this factor at work in our co-therapy relationships. In a group of severely disturbed psychotic adults, Bill's co-therapist, Jim, contributes a frankness and directness of expression to the group that cuts through much of the verbal haze and makes it easier for the patients to mobilize their energies. Although Jim's interventions produce positive results, there are many times when patient–therapist boundaries can be obscured by this method. In that case, both patients and therapist experience a sense of identity confusion. Bill brings firm psychological boundaries to the co-therapy relationship and to the treatment setting, which creates an area of safety where countertransference anxiety can be contained. Bill embodies a sense of appropriateness that is a corrective balance to Jim's sometimes outlandish comments. Yet Jim's comments are often a refreshing break in the tedium and inertia of a psychotic group.

Another example is the co-therapy Vivian and George do with a codependent couple. Whereas Vivian is directive and confrontive with the couple and attempts to guide them through the change process, George makes the couple do more of the work themselves. He is very patient with slow progress and is quite willing to let them stumble through their own impasses while making observations based on his acute intuitive understanding of who they are. Vivian provides a corrective balance in that she will not allow the couple to drift into a hopeless, helpless attitude and will confront them strongly if their actions threaten to bring disaster on themselves.

Bill and Vivian provide a complementary balance for each other in a therapy group for adult men and women who suffer from a variety of personality and anxiety disorders. Bill's irreverent attitude and humorous one-liners are effective gambits to break through personal impasses in which members of the group find themselves from time to time. They laugh and respond with a lightness that undermines their resistance. Vivian's complementary balance is her close attention to detail and fine memory of what each person says. Her gift inspires people's trust in her because they perceive her ability to listen and care. As effective as irreverence and humor are, they become one dimensional and impertinent if persons in treatment fail to feel listened to or cared for. However, the attention to the seriousness of each person's life can become tedious if not gracefully interspersed with levity, irony, and a touch of the absurd.

## COMPATIBILITY OF THEORETICAL VIEWPOINTS

The compatibility of co-therapists' theoretical viewpoints also can be amply demonstrated by our co-therapy experiences. Vivian's theoretical proclivity is toward the individual, and she has studied assiduously Eric Berne's transactional analysis. She emphasizes the capability of a person in either group or individual psychotherapy to analyze and comprehend the many themes and patterns of behavior that make up his or her life script. She believes that once a person is aware of the choices he or she has made in fulfillment of his or her life script, he or she can challenge and eventually change the behavior that supports the script.

Bill emphasizes group process and believes that an individual's personality is a product of social forces, wherein a person must choose among specific actions that support the picture of reality presented by his or her family or community. An individual may stubbornly persist in these actions out of loyalty or consistency to the original family or community even though they are harmful to him- or herself. Bill thinks the change process begins with individual awareness of the choices he or she has made, but both the awareness and the decision to change must be reinforced by practice in a new social setting where approval is given. Bill's accent on the social aspects of behavioral change is different but not contradictory to Vivian's theoretical stance. In the practice of co-therapy, a synthesis of these two systems is accomplished because both therapists are open about the differences and respect each other's choices and theoretical foundations. If, however, they did not share certain assumptions, or their assumptions varied too widely, the achievement of this kind of synthesis would be undermined.

For example, we both believe in the concepts of transference and countertransference. Although we may not always employ them in the treatment of our patients, they remain concepts whose usefulness has been demonstrated to us in clinical practice. If, however, one of us were adamantly opposed to these concepts, it would be difficult for us to fuse our efforts cooperatively, and it would lead to needless confusion in the minds of our patients.

In another example, we both believe in the concept of group process. That means we both recognize the power and influence that the therapy group as a whole exerts over the behavior of the individual in that group. In many ways, we differ on the nature of its power and the degree of its influence, but the concept of group process is shared by both. Quite an incompatible situation exists when one therapist insists on always doing therapy with individuals in the group while his or her co-therapist tries to relate the individual's actions to a larger group phenomenon. This kind of treatment sets up an adversarial situation in which patients have to choose sides between therapists much as they had to choose sides between parents in their families of origin. This is a prime example of co-therapy dysfunction, a topic we discuss in detail in Chapter 5.

However, many serious theoretical disputes can be tolerated if the other criteria for co-therapy success are satisfied. For example, Bill's theoretical foundations allow the therapist to hold and hug clients when physical touching is appropriate for their disorder and requested by them. He worked with a co-therapist whose theoretical orientation discouraged any physical contact between therapists and patients. She respected Bill's knowledge and liked the way he empathized with people. In the context of the groups they co-led, she saw that he established firm psychological boundaries between himself and the clients. Furthermore, she saw that touching was always an option for the client and never an expectation of the therapist. She observed that it had diagnostic value because it was an indicator of how safe the environment had become for group members. Bill liked his co-therapist and respected her ability to communicate openly her disagreement with him. They were able to accommodate each other because he did not judge her rigid for her belief and she did not judge him unprofessional for his.

However, it is difficult to imagine an accommodation between co-therapists who differ radically on certain theoretical issues despite the regard they demonstrate for each other. For example, a therapist who believes that children are to some degree at fault for their sexual abuse by adults will have a hard time co-leading a group of adults sexually abused as children if his or her co-therapist believes that children are not at fault. These beliefs affect the treatment process itself, and each leads to very different ideas and approaches to curing the patients of their suffering. To attempt to conduct co-therapy under such conditions would be simply misguided and probably destructive to the mental health of the clients.

In our experience, major differences in theoretical viewpoints do not preclude a co-therapy relationship if, on balance, other factors emerge as more important to the treatment process. Bill has done co-therapy with behaviorists who do not believe in the unconscious and found it refreshing to see the same family dynamics given a different interpretation. It did not adversely affect the family in treatment because the co-therapists agreed on a certain plan of action and did not discuss theoretical and philosophical differences in the presence of the family or confuse the family with conflicting jargon. Although major theoretical differences do not preclude co-therapy, they do limit how far a co-therapy team can go in the development of their work relationship. The satisfaction of working together is not as great, and the motivation to continue collaboration is not present in the same way.

The final four criteria demonstrate the primacy of the relationship to the success of the co-therapy team. It is possible that a simply fortuitous matching of therapists can yield a complementary balance of skills and a compatibility of theoretical viewpoints. However, it is highly unlikely that fortune alone will engender openness in communication or equality of participation between co-therapists. Similarly, liking and respecting each other as people require effort and attention by both parties.

## OPENNESS IN COMMUNICATION

Openness in communication between co-therapists is put to the test by countertransference, the experience of strong emotions by therapists about the patients they are treating. Openness is tested in two ways. First, one must trust his or her co-therapist to share these strong emotions if they are in one's consciousness. Second, if the co-therapist's strong emotions and unusual behavior are not within his or her consciousness, his or her partner must bring them to his or her attention. The partner must feel trust in how the feedback will be received in order to confront in this way.

For example, Vivian was aware of her judgmental attitudes toward a male client who was addicted to marijuana and had not worked in 12 years. She and George were treating the man in couple therapy, and she realized that she must share these attitudes with her co-therapist. She wanted George to be alert to ways her judgments might break into the course of treatment and interfere with the therapy. George was less judgmental of the client's financial dependency on his wife and was able to listen to Vivian who was highly critical of the dependency. Interestingly, as the therapy progressed, George became increasingly judgmental of the husband's marijuana addiction. He shared his criticisms with Vivian, who by that time was much more accepting of the client. They were able to modulate the level of their criticism of a very difficult patient by open dialogue with each other.

In another example, the authors were treating in co-therapy a borderline patient, Christine, whose treatment we describe in depth in Chapter 6. For a while her therapy consisted of once-a-week group and twice-a-week individual sessions, one session with Bill and the other with Vivian. Originally, Christine had been an individual patient of Bill's, and the arrangement of meeting with each therapist separately was a transitional phase to individual sessions with both therapists in co-therapy. Within the first month, Vivian had twice forgotten her appointment with Christine, a highly unusual event for Vivian. Bill pointed this out and helped her to understand her countertransference. Christine's bond with Bill after 2 years of individual work was strong, and she was reluctant to meet with Vivian. Vivian began her countertransference by feeling left out. Once Vivian became aware of her own emotional response to the fact that Christine cared more for Bill than for her, she could begin the work of establishing her own bond with Christine. Open communication allowed Bill to invite Vivian to look deeper into the unconscious motives of her forgetting.

Another time, Vivian confronted Bill on his indulgence of Christine's manipulation when he offered Christine an individual session following her abrupt departure from a co-therapy session with Bill and Vivian. Vivian pointed out that Bill was reinforcing her regression and acting out by giving her extra time. In doing so, he supported her resistance to making a bond with Vivian. The co-therapists discussed the issue thoroughly between themselves and interpreted the acting out to the patient. Christine reacted emotionally to the interpretation and gained maturity by her insight. A confrontation of this kind is most difficult for a co-therapist to make because it requires that his or her co-therapist be able to listen clearly and not become defensive or possessive of the client in question. Open communication permits feedback and discussion at this level of depth and intimacy.

In group and family therapy, openness in communication can occur at four different levels: (1) as part of the preparation before entering a session; (2) during a session; (3) as part of the post-session review and feedback; and (4) sharing personal life information that may or may not affect the psychotherapy. Most co-therapy teams will confine their

communication to the first three levels. Sharing personal life information is a major focus for co-therapists who have reached Phase 4 of
their co-therapy team development as described by Dugo and Beck.
Teams in this phase have established mutual acceptance and comfort
and spend less time processing their relationship and devote more time
to their patients (see Chapter 7). However, as Dugo and Beck point
out, when co-therapists at any phase of development foresee stressful
events which will impact their work together, they must communicate
them to their partners. Such events include a new marriage, birth of a
child, divorce, health problems and illnesses in the family, financial
difficulties, being sued for malpractice, and the relocation or retirement
from one's practice. Discussions of this sort are part of the life of
married and intimate couples, as Bob and Mary Goulding show in
Chapter 8.

We recommend that co-therapists check out assumptions with each
other as a way to give expression to those intuitive ideas they develop
about each other. If an assumption does not fit, it may prove to be an
interesting revelation of one person's projection onto his or her co-
therapist. Whether the assumption applies or not, it usually leads to
clarification of the co-therapy environment. For example, a therapist
checked out the assumption that her co-leader was angry after a family
session. Her partner denied anger but was aware of fear within himself
about an impending operation on a member of his own family. Further
discussion of this topic proved to be a relief for both therapists.

Just prior to the start of a session, many important signals and
reminders can be shared in open dialogue between co-therapists.
Sometimes Bill will say, "I'm tired tonight," and Vivian will respond,
"OK, I'll be the active one, and you can watch the process." Or
perhaps Vivian will say to Bill, "You've got to stop Claire tonight.
She's monopolizing the session. When I try to intervene, she projects
her mother's face onto me as a controlling witch." Or Bill may recall
how well Vivian handled a particularly hostile client. "I liked the way
you calmed Beth down last week without minimizing the importance
of her anger." Generous stroking and positive acknowledgement of
this kind are especially conducive to keeping lines of communication
open between colleagues.

When co-therapists stroke each other during a session, two goals are
achieved. First, the therapists communicate their sense of pride and
admiration with their partners, and second, they model a method of
positive reinforcement for their clients. For example, Bill will say to
Vivian, "I'm impressed with your ability to remember the dream Len
had 2 months ago. It certainly relates to what he is saying now." Or

Vivian will say to Bill, "That's a good point you're raising with Adelle. She does twist her mouth in a crooked fashion when she speaks of her mother."

Open communication in group sessions can also take the form of disagreements. Vivian may object to Bill's laughter at an inappropriate time, if a client with a "Don't make it" injunction jokes about losing his job. Bill may openly disagree with Vivian's tolerance of Christine returning to a co-dependent relationship at a particularly vulnerable time in her therapy. "I know Christine needs emotional support to get through this period, but is this the best way for her to get it?" Sometimes in group, co-therapists must give instructions or directions to each other. In one session, the group's emotional leader was pre-paring herself to leave group after many years. She acknowledged how deeply attached she was to her father's wish that she remain "his little girl." The group reminded Melanie of her "Don't grow up" injunction (Goulding & Goulding, 1978). Vivian stated directly and openly to Bill, "You must give Melanie permission to leave." The intervention was effective because Vivian invited Bill to become the powerful male therapist with a patient with whom she had a strong transferential bond. Frank communication was the key to its success.

Post-group therapy sessions are critical times for the exchange of perspectives and feelings and strokes between co-therapists. The fol-lowing is a typical exchange:

VIVIAN: I saw Kevin react much more maturely than in the past when he didn't have time to speak. Do you agree?

BILL: Yes, he's more mature. But he still has a hard time listening to others. Next week, let's watch and stroke him when we see him responding to other people's statements.

VIVIAN: You didn't do too well with your attempt to draw Shawn out of her shell. She's a tough one, since she won't respond to humor.

BILL: Not my variety at least. We may have to wait until she begins to identify with the work of others in the group.

VIVIAN: I liked it when you stopped Rob from putting himself down. That worked well, especially since the theme that emerged in group tonight was self-esteem.

BILL: Yes, I agree. But what was happening with Betsy? She keeps her feelings so well hidden. I'm glad you picked up on her anxiety while I was working with Joe.

VIVIAN: Thanks. I think it has to do with her father and his injunction that she not be important, but I'm not sure. Let's return to that next time and probe some more.

BILL: I agree.

VIVIAN: I did have a problem with your reference to me being like your grandfather.

BILL: It did seem relevant to Rob's struggle around making each woman he dates into his father.

VIVIAN: That's true, but it seemed inappropriately intimate. He didn't need to know that information. You could have said men often select masculine traits in women and accomplished the same thing.

BILL: I don't agree but I see your point. I'm sorry you felt I shared too much about us. I'll keep the professional boundaries tighter with him in the future. I said it because I wanted him to feel something.

VIVIAN: You identify with him?

BILL: Quite a bit.

VIVIAN: That's good to know. I can help you monitor for countertransference.

BILL: Speaking of that, you know Rich is in love with you. Do you see that?

VIVIAN: I hadn't thought of it in those terms, but you may be right. It would be very embarrassing for him if we confront him directly with that, especially since he's just starting to work on his sexual identity as a male.

BILL: Exactly. Maybe I can help him understand how much he sees in you, the nurturing mother he never had. Then he can take a little distance from you and feel closer to me. I can help him get close to you in non-seductive ways that are less threatening to him.

VIVIAN: Sounds good. Does that do it for the group?

BILL: I need a hug.

VIVIAN: That sounds good, too.

As our dialogue shows, useful strategies develop during post-treatment sessions that can influence and alter co-therapy conduct in future sessions.

Much of what we say above concerning openness in communication between co-therapists in group psychotherapy can be applied to family therapy and couple therapy sessions as well.


## EQUALITY OF PARTICIPATION

Whereas a complementary balance of skills involves a blending of abilities to match the needs of the treatment setting, equality of participation means fully sharing the authority of leadership. This means that co-therapists share the responsibility of making decisions and being actively engaged. Equality of participation does not mean the same verbal output or performing the same tasks. It does mean the team will divide the labor in a way that makes sense based on who they are as individuals and the needs of their patients. Most co-therapists do not start out as equals in this respect, but they become so over time if their team is to be successful.

Some co-therapists arrange a division of labor from the start to balance the levels of participation. For example, one leader takes responsibility for opening remarks to the group and announcements, and the other leader takes responsibility for ending on time and other aspects of closure. The psychological equation that must be satisfied is simply this: each person must carry his own share of the load, and neither person must feel he or she is being taken advantage of.

In practice, it becomes more complicated. Many emotional factors influence a psychotherapist's willingness to participate. For example, especially resistant or critical clients can arouse verbosity in some therapists. A therapist may begin to talk more in order to win client approval or establish him- or herself as the more powerful healer. Competition to be liked or preferred by a client can also lead to distortions of equality. A therapist may attempt to be "more giving" or "more helpful" to patients than his or her partner. Unfortunately, contention of this kind forces the patients to choose between their therapists much as the patients at one time were forced to choose between their parents.

Equality of participation can vary across modes of treatment. Some therapists may prefer family therapy and demonstrate more confidence in that arena than in group. Their confidence will be expressed by how fully they take part in the family sessions. Also, therapists' degrees of participation will differ from one constellation of clients to the next depending on the members in the group or the family and the clinical tasks specific to each one. Given certain experiences and interests, a therapist may be quite active in a bereavement group yet more subdued in a group for incest survivors. Another therapist may be less active in an alcoholic family than a schizophrenic family. Each co-therapy pair must strive for equality of participation and make this an expressed goal in their contract to be co-therapists.

The level of therapist activity can vary across the phases of development of a psychotherapy group. During the contractual phase, or Phase I of Ariadne Beck's nine phases of group psychotherapy development (see Appendix), Vivian tends to be more active than Bill. During Phase II, a phase of conflict and competition, both Vivian and Bill are quite active. In Phase IV, Bill is very animated pointing out examples of intimacy as they become manifest in the group. By Phase V, the establishment of mutuality, both Vivian and Bill have diminished their own levels of activity. The level of therapist energy will vary also with the type of therapy provided. For example, Bill will usually take the lead in clinical applications of psychodrama and Vivian will come to the fore with interventions involving transactional analysis.

In our initial interviews with patients, we emphasize that both of us are available for individual appointments throughout their course of treatment in co-therapy. We make a special effort in the first interview to talk in equal amounts in order to set the tone for future work. Often Bill will find his competitive instincts ignited by first interviews with males and Vivian must equalize the energy by focusing her attention on the client and his concerns.

The willingness to reveal oneself to one's co-therapist is a cornerstone for equal participation. A fear of this process will block the therapists' natural spontaneity and compromise their ability to be genuine persons in the therapeutic setting. A strong fear of making mistakes will also truncate the mutuality of interaction between therapists at work. In this case, much energy is consumed in self-conscious self-observation, and many opportunities to listen accurately and respond appropriately are missed.

One co-therapist in a team may in fact believe that he or she *is* unequal. This person's experience of inadequacy will color the way in which he or she can fully participate as a co-therapist. In practice, this psychotherapist may defer continually to his or her partner and undermine all attempts to strike an equal balance. To work with persons who believe themselves unequal is not satisfactory for most co-therapists. Either they will seek consultation to amend the imbalance or they will end the relationship.

If one therapist is being open in communication and his or her partner is not, it will always affect equal participation as a team. For example, if a woman therapist does not correct the misstatements of fact by her male co-therapist in the mistaken belief that she must make the male look good, she forfeits her chance to participate equally. They would then be well along the road to becoming a dysfunctional team.

Mutual stroking during a co-therapy session is one way of clearly demonstrating equality. This is a phenomenon that rarely happens between nequipos. Even an advanced student does not presume to stroke his teacher or supervisor during a psychotherapy session, although he or she may do so afterwards. To do so during a session would seem impertinent. A senior therapist, however, will often stroke in this manner in order to increase the confidence of his or her student. The one-way stroking makes explicit their unequal relationship. That is precisely why the teacher's acknowledgment feels so good to the student. The stroke says the student is measuring up to the level of the senior clinician.

Co-therapists must also share equally in clinical decisions. Clients experience their therapists as equals because the decisions that affect them are shared. For example, the clients see their co-therapists discuss and make decisions together in sessions. They also see the results of joint decision making that occurs outside their sessions and feel the cooperative spirit between their therapists. They certainly are aware of the tension that exists between co-therapists when one therapist makes a clinically important decision without consulting the other. The capacity for shared or consensual decision making is critical at this level of success.

## LIKING EACH OTHER

Most successful co-therapists probably like each other. But that may not always be the case. As part of their training, psychotherapists learn how to work with patients whom they may neither like nor respect. They can do this in the setting of psychotherapy because therapists and patients are not equal in the emotional power or authority that they respectively bring to the therapeutic encounter. Because of the special demands of equality that come into play in a relationship between peers, co-therapists must usually like each other in order for them to do the job.

There are exceptions to this rule. A person may choose to study with a particular therapist in order to acquire specific knowledge or a special skill although the person does not view the therapist as "likable." In this case, the desire to learn transcends the need to like. Respect for the therapist's ability becomes the relevant factor.

Ambition can motivate the choice of co-therapist. Some therapists may choose to co-lead with famous or near-famous clinicians simply to advance their own careers. Virginia Satir, in Chapter 9, speaks of this happening to her on several occasions, much to her dismay. A young therapist may attempt to launch a career by riding the "coat-tails" of a well-established therapist by becoming his or her co-therapist. These choices may have little to do with liking each other as people and more to do with flattery, self-aggrandizement, and the exchange of money. It is valid to ask, as the Gouldings do in Chapter 8, "Why do this if you're not having fun?"

Liking someone contributes immensely to the fun of co-therapy. Some therapists may enter the co-therapy relationship in good faith, believing they truly like their partners, only to discover, as many couples in love discover, that they do not like each other after all. For this reason, we recommend a flexible approach to the choice of co-therapists. Don't plan too far in advance with any new co-therapist, but allow the partnership to unfold incrementally. Judgment of whom one likes can be faulty and one's judgment can change over time. To like one's co-therapist does not necessarily mean being friends or socializing. It does mean that they do enjoy each other's company while doing a task of clinical importance and considerable complexity.

## RESPECT

Most successful co-therapists probably respect each other. Still, that may not always be the case. Impaired psychotherapists who have committed acts of sexual misconduct with patients or abused drugs or alcohol lose the respect of their professional colleagues. It is important to recognize that, following rehabilitation, impaired therapists can earn the trust of colleagues that the misbehavior will not be repeated and establish co-therapy relationships with their peers. A lack of respect for the misdeeds of the past is a part of such a relationship, but so is the expectation that the rehabilitated therapist will not lie and abuse the therapy relationship in the here and now. A person may be liked and valued for whoever he or she is in the present although not respected for what he or she has done in the past.

One can respect the knowledge and experience of a therapist and not like him or her as a person. An example is the able and talented psychotherapist who is highly narcissistic. One can respect a marginally astute psychotherapist because of his or her efforts to overcome personal suffering and emotional handicaps. One can respect the expertise of a fine clinician and dislike his or her critical tongue. However, the prospects for a long-term, mutually satisfying, and functional co-therapy team developing from such a match are questionable.

## THE SUCCESSFUL CO-THERAPY TREATMENT
## OF A MARRIED COUPLE

To demonstrate the successful application of these factors in clinical practice, we offer the following couple whom we treated in conjoint marital therapy. Marjorie and Ivan had known each other for six years and had been married for two years when they were referred to treatment. Ivan had two teenage sons from his first marriage, one of whom was in recovery for drug addiction. Both sons were living with them and were a stimulus for much uproar between husband and wife. The course of couple therapy was moderately successful and extended for 30 sessions across one year.

The presenting problem was conflict concerning how the teenagers were going to be disciplined and how the parents were going to set limits. Marjorie wanted appreciation for the work she did in setting limits with the children. At the same time, she resented Ivan's inaction and avoidance of problems of discipline when they emerged. Ivan wanted his wife to calm down and be less anxious and to stop nagging him. He also wanted her to be less dependent emotionally on him because her self-esteem suffered if she did not receive his recognition.

We perceived the following cycle of pathological communication in which either partner could start the process. Marjorie became hurt and angry when Ivan withdrew and withheld affection from her. She expresssed anger. Ivan became afraid and withheld affection even more. Ivan perpetuated the cycle as much with his fear as Marjorie did with her anger.

Both partners exhibited codependent behavior. Ivan neglected to enforce rules with his sons in an effort to obtain their approval by being "Mr. Nice Guy." His behavior enraged Marjorie, who came off as the "bitch" when she confronted his co-dependency. He would say he was "hurt," and Marjorie was left to act out the anger for both. Marjorie did not believe she was intelligent and needed Ivan's acknowledgment, which he withheld when he was angry or withdrawn.

The co-therapy strategy for this couple involved accurate diagnosis of both the man's and woman's individual dynamics and the treatment of their individual pathology in couple therapy. We diagnosed the couple as a passive, mildly depressed male and a histrionic female who both demonstrated poor communication skills, a recurring motif in many marriages. Marjorie had been put down by her alcoholic father. Bill's special attention to stroke her intelligence and determination helped to heal that wound. Both therapists stroked her for her intuitive abilities and her enthusiasm. As an only child of emotionally ungiving parents, Ivan learned to be controlling with his mother. "If I didn't take control with her, she would have smothered me," he said. In his attempts to control Marjorie, Ivan confused her with his mother. Vivian helped Ivan see how Marjorie was different in that he could listen to Marjorie *and* he could talk about what he wanted. Marjorie experienced Ivan as controlling. She confused him with her father, who was a tyrant. Both spouses had controlling parents, and they brought those memories into their relationship with each other.

Ivan became very angry at Marjorie and did not express it directly. "I don't feel safe expressing my anger with her because it escalates," he said. Much effort was expended encouraging his direct expression of resentment in the therapy sessions, especially concerning her hugging and kissing him when he was angry or upset, because he perceived her actions as attempts to manipulate him.

Because of the degree of anger, hostility, and distrust, it would have been very difficult to work with this couple as a solo therapist. As co-therapists, we looked forward to working together and brought our joyful anticipation to each session despite the acrimonious atmosphere in the early stage of treatment. We could formulate a more positive prognosis because we were encouraged by our own experience as a couple who had worked through similar impasses. We passed along our encouragement to the embattled pair.

In the beginning they were not pleasant to work with. Neither Ivan nor Marjorie was particularly likable since they both assumed defensive postures that were egocentric and self-absorbed. As co-therapists we shared with them how we liked each other as partners. This played a major role in the couple's treatment. We shared how different we were as people and how we appreciated our differences and did not criticize our distinctiveness. This helped them to see that personality differences did not mean incompatibility. We taught them couple communication exercises, such as George Bach's creative uses of aggression to foster intimacy: Resentments and Appreciations, Vesuvius, and Checking Out Assumptions (Bach & Wyden, 1970). We never asked them to do a task that we did not first complete ourselves in their presence. We walked them through several fights in order to teach them the skills of fighting fairly. Practicing these skills increased their ability to listen better and express their needs directly.

As their needs became known, they emerged from their defensive postures and became more likable. They became cute with one another in their expressions of affection. A turning point came when Vivian helped Ivan realize that he did not have to solve Marjorie's problems. Vivian gave him a homework asssignment to remind himself of Marjorie's statement in the session, "I am responsible for my own happiness." Ivan discovered that he needed only to listen to Marjorie's problems. Furthermore, Bill gave Ivan permission to express anger at her directly. With encouragement, Ivan said "no" to Marjorie's request that he give up his many church meetings where he received much recognition. He also disagreed openly with Marjorie's desire to reduce their financial support for his oldest child who had moved out on his own. His confidence grew as he discovered that his negative feelings did not produce catastrophes for the marriage. To his surprise, Marjorie was able to trust him more because he was being honest and direct. She was less lonely because he did not withdraw so much emotionally. Ivan's anger was no longer expressed as condescending remarks, which had so irritated Marjorie because they reminded her of her father.

Another turning point in the treatment occurred when Bill pointed out to Ivan how he deprived himself of his wife's company by withdrawing and not listening to her needs. In this way, he perpetuated the loneliness of his childhood. This intervention made an impact on Ivan and helped him see how he depressed himself. Bill also helped Ivan realize that he had been depriving himself of the experience of his own feelings of love. This realization affected him profoundly and led to further behavior change.

The primary work of the co-therapy team centered on instruction about intimacy and communication. We modeled corrective couple communication from the start by giving each other positive strokes. We became very active early in the course of treatment, sharing the job of pointing out to Marjorie when she became a tyrant like her father. We became active in pushing Ivan to speak and act in ways congruent with his feelings. Both therapists were equally involved in these activities.

Private consultations between the co-therapists played a major role in the treatment of this couple. In our strategy sessions, we planned that Vivian would back off when Marjorie transferred onto Vivian the negative feelings she experienced for her father. Bill would intervene and analyze Marjorie's transference to Vivian and help her talk about what she really needed as a child in her abusive family of origin.

Both co-therapists were gratified because the presence of a partner in the same room prevented countertransference from becoming an obstacle to the therapy. Vivian could understand and identify with Marjorie's anger at a withholding male. Vivian was impatient to have Marjorie become more loving as she herself had done. Bill helped her with her impatience. Bill could understand and identify with Ivan's anger and withdrawal in the face of a histrionic female. Bill was impatient to have Ivan become more assertive, as he had done. Vivian helped him with his impatience. Neither Bill nor Vivian could have been as effective alone as they were as a team.

In retrospect, we believe Vivian could not have been successful alone, since her attempts to nurture Ivan would have appeared like betrayal to Marjorie. This is a distinct advantage the co-therapy team enjoys over the solo therapist. Also, Marjorie's excessive verbalizations had to be stopped. When Vivian attempted to stop her, Marjorie experienced it as a rejection from her father. Marjorie had to be stopped and needed someone to recognize her feelings at the time. Bill was able to do that simply by giving her strokes like, "You don't have to go on and on. I believe you're smart." Because of Vivian's presence, Bill was better able to listen to Marjorie and to empathize with her. The sum total of our co-therapeutic efforts provided Ivan with safety to express anger and allowed Marjorie to feel listened to in their couple sessions.

Many couples seek us as a co-therapy team. We believe there are distinct advantages afforded by the co-therapy approach with couples. The couples who enter treatment with us come with a sense of positive expectation. They believe each will be heard better. They assume we can communicate better than they. They believe we can cooperate better than they. They assume they can learn from us.

## THE SUCCESSFUL CO-THERAPY TREATMENT OF A FAMILY

Harold was a banking executive in northern California who presented himself and his much younger second wife, Julie, to Bill in their initial couple therapy session with the words, "We'd like you to solve a problem for us." They were both concerned with the way Harold's son, Wilbur, was treating his stepmother. "He rejects me and makes our life together miserable," said Julie in describing her nineteen-year-old stepson. Harold carried himself with a military bearing and, although 25 years older than his psychotherapist, addressed Bill as "sir." Harold had been a Navy pilot in the battle for Tarawa in the South Pacific during the Second World War, and he had earned a Silver Star for valor in prolonged, intense combat conditions. He had been divorced from his first wife for eight years, and Wilbur was the youngest of their three sons. Julie, his new wife of two years, was the mother of three grown children herself and had divorced her first husband about the same time she married Harold. Wilbur lived with his father and stepmother while he attended classes at the university. His own mother had remarried and moved to New York shortly after her divorce from Harold. Following the initial session, they agreed to enter family therapy with Wilbur.

In their first conjoint session, Wilbur presented as a good-looking young man who was taller than his father and had solemn but piercing blue eyes. He wanted Julie to move out and have Dad for himself, and he said so directly. Harold wanted Julie to accept Wilbur and not fight so much. He loved both his son and Julie but felt anguish that he was being asked to choose between them. Julie wanted Wilbur to respect her and obey the rules of the house, which included cleaning up the kitchen and picking up the art supplies that he left everywhere. Wilbur challenged her every criticism with an impertinent remark, "It's not your house, it's my father's house!"

Harold was tolerant and indulgent of his son to the extreme. He would promise Julie that he would "crack down" on Wilbur only to be more permissive than before, which inspired her to new heights of fury. It was Julie's intense anger that prompted Bill to seek the support of a female co-therapist, Yvonne, as a buffer to help stem the overt hostility between stepmother and son and balance the male–female energy in the family treatment. Bill had worked with Yvonne as his co-therapist with quite a few families in family therapy over 3 years. She possessed strong analytic skills, good clinical judgment, and the capacity to nurture appropriately. He was grateful that she could join him in treating this family.

BILL: So, from what I've told you, what do you think?

YVONNE: Reminds me of the O'Shaunnessy family.

BILL: That bad! Of course, that was a couple of years ago, and we didn't know each other that well. We've learned a few things since then.

YVONNE: What's the family secret?

BILL: I don't know. But with your help, we'll find out.

In their first co-therapy treatment session, Julie opened with complaints of Wilbur's "sullen" attitude and "sloppy" personal traits. "Wilbur doesn't have any friends," she contended. "All he does is mope around the house and make a mess." She accused Wilbur of trying to drive her away from the home, and she threatened to leave Harold if he didn't do something about it now. Both father and son remained impassive as she spoke, Wilbur looking distractedly out of the window and Harold looking directly at his wife with something like a noncomprehending stare. Yvonne did much of the therapeutic work in these early sessions, empathically allowing Julie to vent her frustrations while all the males, including Bill, remained silent. She gently questioned Julie about what her expectations had been when she had first met and married Harold, subtly pointing out that Harold had been taking care of Wilbur with a modicum of success six full years before she had entered upon the scene. Yvonne was able to make a bond with the narcissistically wounded child within Julie across the course of ten to twelve family sessions. She established herself as a nurturing mother for Julie while the males appeared ineffectual in their attempts to change the despairing and negatively charged mood within the family.

It became clear to Bill that both the father and son were severely depressed, and as Yvonne treated Julie's narcissistic disturbance, he began to focus steadily on the lack of affect the males demonstrated. "The only time you two laugh," Bill interjected, "is when Julie makes some clearly outrageous and provocative exclamation." This interpretation explored the purpose both father and son found in Julie's presence: a source of relief for the unending sorrow in which both lived. But why such sorrow?

Yvonne and Bill discussed the family after each encounter and were divided about how to proceed with treatment. Yvonne believed she should treat Julie separately to focus on her underlying issues, and Bill believed they should continue treating the family as a unit, exploring ways to maintain its integrity. By the fifteenth family session, Julie had moved to a house she owned in the same town, creating another crisis for the family. Yvonne began treating Julie in individual therapy and also continued her co-therapy treatment of father and son. In the first session with Julie absent, Wilbur appeared to gloat in his victory of removing the unwanted stepmother from the family. Harold, however, was panicked that Julie was gone and would never come back to him. He began to ruminate about the many losses he had sustained in his life, referring now to his days at war, a subject he had kept closely hidden in the face of the therapists' frequent inquiries. As the father spoke more of his war experiences, his son appeared visibly deflated as if he were reliving the events himself. Drawing on her intuition, Yvonne interjected a masterful, "These stories aren't new to you, are they Wilbur?" Her question seemed to touch him deeply and drove his father deeper into reflections about his special relationship with his son.

Before the next visit, Wilbur made a suicide gesture, slashing his jugular vein superficially with his father's razor. Bill began the next co-therapy session with the query, "Why the razor?" Harold explained the special significance of the razor. It was the gift of his wartime buddy for whom Wilbur was named, a buddy who had died in the first terrible days of the Tarawa invasion. Wilbur left the session abruptly as his father spoke of the war. Bill followed him outside, leaving Yvonne to explore further the father's memories of war traumas. During this extended session, which lasted two and one-half hours, Bill sat and talked quietly to Wilbur, who wavered between silent withdrawal and agitated shaking and sudden bursts of speech. Wilbur demonstrated all the classic signs of post-traumatic stress syndrome, including detailed flashbacks about experiences he obviously took no direct part in but learned only as story fragments from his father. At these moments, Wilbur tended to take on aspects of his father's personality, appearing much older and speaking in a deeper voice.

All participants of this particular family session were drained emotionally at its conclusion. Yvonne and Bill discussed afterwards their next move.

YVONNE: Perhaps we should continue one on one with each of them. There's so much individual pathology to uncover.

BILL: Sure, there's plenty of pathology, but we've got to confront the suicide stuff first. We've got to help the boy differentiate from his dad—and we can do that best in conjoint sessions.

YVONNE: Let's get the father to talk about his best friend, Wilbur, and keep the son in session to ask questions about his namesake.

In the subsequent hour, Yvonne probed the father's memories of his friend while Bill supported Wilbur's staying in the session to listen not just to the story but to his father's feelings. At one point, Harold produced an old snapshot of his buddy and burst into tears, mourning the loss deeply. Wilbur watched his father in rapt fascination and said later, "I've never seen him cry." He put his hand on his father's shoulder and said with tears in his eyes, "I don't want to be like you. You've got no friends. All of your friends died in the war. I'm very lonely, and I want to have friends."

His father appeared dumbfounded, shaking his head repeatedly and uttering softly, "I didn't know, I didn't know." He expressed again and again how he wanted his son to live and be happy and to have companions. Both men embraced at the close of the session.

Following this breakthrough, Julie was brought back to family therapy, and gradually the insights the men had uncovered began to be integrated into the family's understanding. Julie shared her own unresolved grief stored up from the untimely death of her father when she was a teenager. She had carried anger for years as a substitute for mourning. All family members drew closer to each other as the healing of bereavement softened the previously sharp edges of their interpersonal conflicts. Bill and Yvonne began the treatment of Julie and Harold as a couple, and Bill continued individual work with Wilbur. The co-therapy treatment of the family had come to an end.

All of the examples given in this chapter illustrate the complexity of how a co-therapy team becomes successful. In the next two chapters, we look deeper at the ways the co-therapy team can exhibit difficulties and the creative ways co-therapists can solve problems in order to facilitate clinical success.

# • 5 •

# *Co-Therapy Teams in Trouble:*
# *Impasses and Crises*

Co-therapy teams face a number of problems with varying degrees of severity from the predictable crises and occasional dilemmas of every team to the systematically flawed operation of a dysfunctional team. Many of these problems can be anticipated by co-therapists, and indeed that is the purpose of Dugo and Beck's model of co-therapy team development in Chapter 7. Armed with some knowledge of what is to come, co-therapists can overcome obstacles and avoid future pitfalls. We intend by this chapter to help teams in trouble face their difficulties and, in some cases, prevent their descent into unnecessary dissolution or frank dysfunction.

When co-therapy teams encounter impasses or crises in their relationships, there are a number of steps they can take to remedy the situation. First, they must become aware that they are troubled and acknowledge to themselves how it affects them and their clients. They may be able to resolve their dilemmas by taking direct action, perhaps consulting this volume, and devoting time and energy to the problem at hand. They may also want to seek external consultation. A team may become dysfunctional as a consequence of their difficulties if they do not follow these steps and, remaining in denial, do damage to themselves and their clients. Teams that become dysfunctional probably will not resolve their issues without help in the form of direct intervention by consultants, supervisors, or knowledgeable peers. Another responsible choice for dysfunctional teams is the agreement to terminate work together. It is the hallmark of skillful and experienced co-therapists to know when they have reached an impasse and to summon the resources to extricate themselves from difficulties.

When co-therapists mishandle the practice of co-therapy within the treatment setting, they run the risk of becoming a dysfunctional team. Several of these offenses are mentioned by the respondents to our survey under the heading of "hazards" in the practice of co-therapy. We shall illuminate these points by examples of co-therapy teams that have become troubled in the treatment of patients.

## DEFINITION OF A DYSFUNCTIONAL TEAM

We want to maintain the useful distinction between the disadvantages of co-therapy that speak to the practical difficulties of co-leading, such as time and money constraints, and the misuse of co-therapy that sabotages the psychotherapy process itself and compromises the integrity and effectiveness of psychotherapists.

Co-therapy dysfunction encompasses more than mistakes committed by co-therapists. Dysfunction implies a systematic failure of the co-therapists either to perform as a treatment team or to communicate as colleagues, or both. A dysfunctional pair will produce negative results for patients and headaches for themselves. Often the patients will be forced to give up what they want and nonverbally embrace a "no-change" contract in which they tacitly agree that they will not make the changes they want while in treatment with this particular co-therapy pair. All co-therapy teams make mistakes in psychotherapy, but a dysfunctional team makes mistakes from which its members by themselves cannot recover. Most often they do not recognize or acknowledge their mistakes. Functional co-therapy teams will make mistakes and be aware of them either at the time or later in discussion with themselves or their consultant. They have the sort of relationship that allows them to work through a mistake of clinical judgment or behavior, face the problem directly, and develop a plan to prevent repetition in the future. We discuss several of our own mistakes as clinicians and co-therapists in Chapter 6.

A dysfunctional co-therapy team—like a dysfunctional family—is often oblivious to its most egregious behavior and may, in fact, exist in complete denial of its faults. The functional co-therapy dyad not only perceives its weaknesses but also anticipates the development of problems that logically result from them. For example, the co-therapy team that strongly wishes to avoid conflict with its patients can predict that the team will encounter particularly difficult times during Phases II and V of Ariadne Beck's phases of group therapy development (Appendix).

Such a team can encourage each other to listen to the anger that smolders just beneath the surface and prepare for inevitable testing by patients.

Many of the examples that we give below are co-therapists facing predictable dilemmas in the developmental process of the co-therapy team. A few of our examples portray dysfunctional teams, some of whom sought help and some that did not. It is difficult for us as clinicians to see ourselves as being part of a troubled team just as it is difficult for us to admit when we do not serve our patients well. As you read this chapter, we recommend that you assume an attitude of one who wants more information and who wants to learn better the practice of a complex skill.

## CO-THERAPISTS IN SUPERVISION

Supervision of a co-therapist team, when a suitable supervisor is available, is always a good idea and should never be considered a failure or weakness on the part of co-therapists who seek it. Many of the problems discussed in this chapter might have been anticipated sooner and with less distress for therapists and patients if co-therapy supervision had been initiated. The following guidelines have proved helpful for supervisors requested to assist co-therapists.

1. Help the co-therapists to clarify the terms of their working contract.
2. Provide a theoretical model of how co-therapy teams work, for example, the six factors for co-therapy success discussed in Chapter 4.
3. Model congruence. Be frank about what you know and what you don't know.
4. Encourage direct communication.
5. Discourage one-upsmanship and unnecessary competition.
6. If the supervision has been required by a superior, make clear to the therapists the consequences of the supervision in terms of job performance rating and evaluation. Are promotions or jobs on the line?
7. Acknowledge the co-therapists equally and recognize the different strengths each brings to the treatment setting.
8. Let them know that they can deepen their work affiliation if they choose to do so.

## CO-THERAPY SUPERVISION WITH ADA AND JERRY

The attitude of the co-therapists in supervision is markedly different when the supervision is required by the boss rather than requested by both therapists. Bill supervised a co-therapy team as part of his job as coordinator for a mental health program. The chief of mental health had approached Bill to carry out the supervision after Ada had complained to the chief that she "could not stand to work with Jerry anymore." Together they were conducting family therapy with six families and co-led one group for substance abusers. As often is the case when one co-therapist initiates a complaint about the other in an institutional setting, Jerry seemed oblivious to Ada's grievances although she claimed to have confronted him often during the 6 months they had worked as a team. They shared equal power administratively and equal responsibility clinically as the only two members of their department. Consequently, their collaboration was absolutely necessary for the functioning of the department. Ada wanted Jerry replaced, not supervisory sessions with him. Jerry wanted to avoid the conflict entirely. Although both co-therapists resented Bill's involvement as a supervisor, their motivation for change was high, since both of their jobs were in jeopardy.

In Bill's first supervisory session with them Ada attacked Jerry for being so passive in their family sessions, particularly with substance-abusing males. Jerry remained silent in the face of her attacks, defending himself from time to time with the statement, "I'm sorry you feel that way." By the end of the session Bill obtained an agreement from both to examine their roles as co-therapists in the sense of the specific tasks they took responsibility for in the clinical setting. It was clear that they shared administrative tasks well, but their work with patients suffered.

In subsequent supervisory sessions Bill supported Jerry's attempts to state his case to Ada. His experience as an officer in the military had taught him to be suspicious of dissent, and he viewed Ada's criticism of him as a kind of insubordination, although they were clearly equals on the organizational chart. When questioned about this Jerry stated emphatically, "I have some things I don't like about her, too, you know." Ada said that she didn't know and this was the first she had heard of any complaints. The team began to share how they viewed each other's interventions in family therapy. Jerry was uncomfortable with the degree of confrontation Ada used in their sessions with families and often believed she conducted herself in an "unladylike" manner. Ada was angry at Jerry's failure to challenge the husbands' behavior in the parenting of the children. She wanted him to be more directive especially in cases where the fathers were being emotionally abusive to their offspring. Jerry agreed that their behavior had to be confronted but seemed at a loss about how to do it.

It was clear that although they were equally competent as individual therapists, Ada held the upper hand in her confidence and skills as a family therapist. Supervisors often consult with co-therapists who are unequal in their skills and participation. Bill encouraged the co-therapists to balance the inequality by a series of experiments whereby Jerry assumed Ada's typical role in sessions and Ada assumed Jerry's. Both therapists reported that they were extremely uncomfortable doing so but also reported some favorable results in the treatment of their families. One family member stated that she had renewed hope in the possibility for people to change because she had witnessed such change in her co-therapists. One child was surprised when Jerry raised his voice to her father, and subsequently her school attendance improved.

By their experiments with role flexibility, the co-therapists were able to strike a balance in their working relationship. Their direct communication had improved considerably, and they were able to acknowledge the strengths each brought to the clinical encounter. Ada acknowledged Jerry's patience and nonjudgmental attitude in his treatment of character-disordered individuals. Jerry acknowledged Ada's clinical assertiveness and sensitive intuition. The co-therapists had used their supervision well in overcoming their crisis to become a co-equal team.

## THE FIVE C'S OF CO-THERAPY DILEMMAS

### Competition

Excessive and unnecessary competition between co-therapists was perceived as the most threatening hazard by our respondents. Since some kinds of competition can prove both healthy and functional, this is a complicated issue that deserves careful analysis. Battles for turf and expressions of territoriality signify co-therapists that are insecure about the boundaries between themselves and the relative value of their respective skills. For example, a team may contend for the title of "best therapist" or "best group therapist" or "best family therapist." These are empty struggles for recognition that leave the contenders impoverished. Both therapists must feel stroked and acknowledged by their collaboration. The joyous pronouncement at the start of the caucus race in Lewis Carroll's *Alice in Wonderland* must apply to co-therapists: "Everybody wins and all must have prizes!" Co-therapists must learn to channel their competition in healthy directions that contribute to their own development and to that of their team. A dialogue along these lines would go as follows:

ALICE: I want to experiment with my ability to confront the denial in our family tonight.

TED: That's a good idea, but only if I do it. You stumble around too much with your words.

ALICE: That's why I need practice, Ted.

TED: Why not stick with family script analysis? That's what you do best.

ALICE: Because I want to expand my repertoire. I think it will strengthen our work together. Does that threaten you?

TED: No, but getting tough verbally has been my trademark. I'll have to back off to let you do the job. That won't be easy for me.

ALICE: Fine. You can still take the lead with them when it comes time for them to confront termination issues. I have no desire to challenge you in that area. That's your forte.

TED: You've got a deal.

Acknowledging the existence of competition opens the possibility for compromise and growth in the team.

Another kind of competition is a rivalry for who will be more important in the life of the patient or in the lives of the group or family members. In group therapy, Dugo and Beck see this phenomenon as a part of a phase of co-therapy development (see Phase 2, Chapter 7) that must be worked through before meaningful co-therapy treatment can begin. Sometimes, however, an experienced co-therapy pair will also face jealousy over who shall possess the lion's share of the positive transference. For example, Vivian once had to leave the group with a coughing spell when Christine discussed how much she missed her close bond with Bill since she began growing closer to Vivian. This unconscious reaction by Vivian was noted and commented on by both therapists. Christine felt gratified that her shift of emotional energy from a father object to a mother object had such impact on her therapists. She also felt relieved that we appreciated how difficult the transition had been for her—although it represented a natural progression in her work with us. We shall speak more of Christine in the next chapter.

An example not only of excessive competition but also of unethical behavior was the case in which the co-therapist stole the client away from his partner. A well-to-do person was referred to a group led by a male–female co-therapy team, and after a while, it became clear that the client needed more than group therapy in order to address his pathology. Without conferring with his co-therapist, the male therapist insisted that the client enter individual treatment with him. He spoke with the client directly in group and gave him no choice of how to proceed with his own treatment. The female co-therapist was appalled but did not confront her co-leader until after group. The male therapist conceded that he had been heavy-handed in the way he offered the client no other alternatives but succeeded in pacifying his co-therapist. Within 2 weeks, however, the male therapist had convinced the client to drop group entirely and enter individual treatment with him alone three times per week. Once again, he had done this without consulting his co-therapist, who was outraged by his behavior. She insisted that they dissolve their co-therapy relationship because of the bad faith he had shown in their work together. He agreed to dissolution of their work contract but on the condition that he take their entire group into his own private practice. What ensued was a bitter struggle for "possession" of the group that eventually destroyed it and damaged several of its members.

The acrimony and passive aggression of this case are extreme, but it points up some important ethical questions for the practice of co-therapy. Who "owns" the client? And who determines if the client needs solo individual treatment and with whom? These are issues many co-therapists would like to side-step, but they do so at the peril of their work relationship. Our bias in favor of equality dictates that each therapist share equally in the responsibility of planning treatment for the patient according to his or her needs and choices. Our approach stresses that the patient must choose autonomously from among treatment alternatives that are most appropriate to his or her condition. Co-therapists must not allow either the convenience or the financial profit of either practitioner to become the determining factor. Co-therapists who drift into that practice will undo their work contract with greed and mistrust. When appropriate, it is most gracious to suggest that a person in co-therapy treatment consider solo work with one's partner. Such a gesture accomplishes two goals: it strokes one's partner, and it conveys one's confidence in him or her to the client. Both are essential in order to maintain a healthy co-therapy contract.

Other symptoms of co-therapist rivalry include cutting off your co-therapist in the middle of his or her statements and making derogatory or negative comments about the suggestions offered by your co-therapist. Disparagement of your partner's idea is not simply disagreement; it is disagreement without ackowledgment of the idea's merit or your partner's good will in offering it. This is a discount of your co-therapist. Virginia Satir gives an excellent example of it in Chapter 9, page 217.

Another more subtle expression of rivalry is inappropriate humor at the expense of your co-therapist. For example, a therapist who makes fun of his or her partner's interpretation of a patient's dream is either expressing hostility indirectly or dueling to be right or both. If put-downs like this are permitted to flower, clients will become increasingly uncomfortable and probably leave treatment prematurely. The co-therapy relationship will deteriorate rapidly no matter how "humorous" or clever the wisecracks.

Power struggles between co-therapists are another form of competition. They usually center around three questions:

1. How will decisions be made?
2. Who will talk and who will be silent and when?
3. Will conflicts be resolved or avoided?

The first involves decision making. The co-therapy contract implies joint decision making, and departures from this practice must be few if trust is to prevail. If a co-therapist unilaterally makes a decision affecting a patient's treatment without consulting his or her partner, an abuse of power has occurred. Veteran co-therapists might protest that they could never do this. But the temptation to do so is always present even among the experienced co-therapists who have achieved the more advanced phases of co-therapists' development described by Dugo and Beck (Chapter 7).

Another example of unilateral decision making is the choice by a therapist to schedule a solo appointment with a person or family without prior consultation with his or her co-therapist. The therapist may be responding to a patient or family in crisis, or he or she may truly believe a session alone with them could prove helpful. Either way, the co-therapy relationship is plunged into conflict by such a maneuver. The course of treatment is called into question as well, since many issues pertinent to treatment are not being addressed. Did the co-therapist offer the extra session or was it requested? If this is a manipulation by the patient, what purpose did he or she hope it would serve? What is the countertransference issue for the therapist involved? The therapists are not taking full advantage of the mutual consultation that co-therapy makes possible. There may be times when solo appointments are indicated for patients in co-therapy treatment. Unavailability of the co-therapist for reasons of illness or vacation or scheduling difficulties are three such cases. The contingencies on which such a decision is based must be resolved beforehand and discussed with the patients as a mutual agreement between therapists. Patients deserve to know the reason why their co-therapists are not treating them as a team.

Co-therapists can also fight over who is "more worthy" to make a particular decision. For example, one therapist may claim preeminence in the determination of a question because of degree, special training, years of experience, books written, or "the patient was my referral in the first place." This is usually a psychological game of "one-upsmanship" and does not help the co-therapy team establish a mutually acceptable protocol for making decisions of clinical import. If a clinician believes he cannot share decision making because of his or her specialized skills, perhaps he or she should reconsider why he or she has chosen to practice co-therapy. There are cases in which decisions are beyond the scope of practice of a particular clinician, as with nonphysicians who cannot prescribe psychotropic medications. In such circumstances, the physician co-therapist will do well to make his or her case for medicating or not medicating and present it as an option to be considered by the team. It is always imcumbent on the person who possesses the specialized knowledge to implement it without patronizing his or her partner or upsetting the equilibrium of the relationship.

The second kind of power struggle involves the amount of talk each will do and when it is appropriate for one or the other to remain silent. When both co-therapists believe the amount of talking each is doing in a therapy session is satisfactory, there is no problem. However, when one therapist resents the degree of participation by his or her co-therapist, because of either silence or overactivity, a problem exists. In Chapter 8 (p. 205), Bob and Mary Goulding characterize this dilemma as the passive–aggressive problem. They observe that the relationship too often degenerates into a contest of blaming the other: "If it weren't for my co-therapist, I'd be (more, less) active." Since equality of participation is listed fourth in our criteria for co-therapy success, a resolution of the conflict is critical for the life of the team.

Therapists can easily fool themselves during the selection of a co-therapist by minimizing the issue of participation. This is unfortunate because the ability to be equal in power is a highly desired trait in co-therapists, and in the treatment setting, the degree and kind of participation by a therapist translates into power. For example, Bill once chose a colleague to co-lead a group with him. He liked her intelligence, genuineness, and curiosity about people. He experienced her openness in their dialogues and found her refreshingly non-rigid and compatible with his own theories of change and growth. Although she was a novice in group therapy, she was eager to learn. Once in group, however, she became silent. At the beginning, this did not trouble Bill, since she seemed to be watching and listening intently. In post-group sessions, she made astute comments, but in group she remained silent. After several months, Bill began to experience loneliness in group. It became clear to him that he wanted companionship in the group, a peer with whom he could interact. When he told her this, she seemed surprised by his expectation and said that was not how she chose to act in a group. She would answer questions when asked directly, but rarely would she offer an observation or initiate an action. Bill's irritation with her grew. The group members appeared oblivious to her inactivity. Bill's interest in the group process itself waned, and he focused his energy on what he could do to make his co-therapist act the way he wanted her to. Both therapists were locked into a passive-aggressive impasse and did not seek consultation to resolve it. Their post-group sessions became brief. Attendance in the group fell off. They waited for the time-limited group mercifully to come to an end.

The example above illustrates how two well-motivated therapists can enter into a co-therapy contract in good faith, only to watch themselves become dysfunctional because they did not make clear the level of activity they expected of each other.

The third kind of power struggle involves whether conflicts will be resolved or avoided. In the conflict above, both Bill and his co-therapist chose to avoid resolution of their difficulty, although that choice was never verbalized or discussed in those terms. However, what happens when one co-therapist wants to seek consultation to face a problem and his or her partner is unwilling? Or suppose one co-therapist wants her partner to read this book and he refuses? What is her recourse?

This dilemma is similar to the intransigence of a therapist who insists on doing the therapy his or her way and is unwilling to discuss it further. For example, the chief of a mental health clinic was co-leading a group of heterosexual couples with a highly competent nurse practitioner. They possessed equal skills clinically and had worked before in other groups as an effective team. However, the chief, a male, laughed spontaneously each time the women in the group suggested that their husbands ought to help with kitchen chores because they were working wives. His laughter greatly irritated his co-therapist, who was female, and yet, she could not impress on him the seriousness of her complaint or the disparaging message he was sending the women in the group. He maintained that she was reading meaning into his behavior that simply was not there. Both agreed that in all other

respects, their collaboration was laudatory. The female therapist requested consultation for the co-therapy team, and the male refused. As
chief of the clinic, he believed it would be a waste of clinic time to go
into consultation with a third party to resolve what he considered to be
a "nonexistent problem." He also expressed the fear that as a result of
the consultation he would be forced to give up an essential part of his
sense of humor. At a stalemate, they both tried to avoid the conflict.
The atmosphere of the co-therapy relationship became tense and the
willingness of couples in the group to reveal about themselves diminished. Finally, after several weeks, a member of the group spoke
directly to the therapists: "I have the sense that you two have something to resolve, and we're not going to move forward until you do."
That statement broke the impasse for a co-therapy team that had
become dysfunctional, and they began a course of reconciliation with
the help of a peer.

The felicitous outcome described above came about because of a
patient's perceptive observation. The request for consultation itself had
evoked strong resistance in the male therapist and surprised his co-
therapist. As co-leaders, they had always functioned well and had
demonstrated much flexibility in resolving disputes. The prospect of
third-party mediation exposed a layer of insecurity in their relationship that had been carefully hidden or had simply not been noticed by
either one. As a rule, any request for peer consultation should be
honored by a co-therapist. If it is an attempt to manipulate the co-
therapy, then this will be revealed during the consultation. It should
not be considered a penalty to be endured for bad behavior, but rather
as a prerequisite for two people trying to share a difficult task.

Therapists may not be excessively competitive and still find themselves in conflict with their co-therapists. When such a conflict lingers
and remains unresolved over time, the fabric of the co-therapy relationship starts to unravel. Each time a therapist challenges the authority or knowledge or behavior of a co-therapist, the opportunity
for conflict arises. Such confrontations can have beneficial outcomes in
terms of new learning and new perspectives for the team. However,
one can anticipate that resentments and recurring feuds will flourish if
the methods of confrontation and peer consultation are not agreed on
and employed.

### Countertransference

Countertransference is clearly not a phenomenon specific to co-
therapy but is possible in all forms of psychotherapy. We maintain that
a co-therapist often can help a partner identify his or her countertrans-

ference as it appears. A problematic situation will occur, however, when neither co-therapist is aware of countertransference as it occurs or perhaps just one is aware and hesitates to call it into question. All of the clinicians in the following examples were bright, astute, and ethically conscious. Their lapses into unconscious behavior were clear to them after the fact but were not visible to them at the time.

Co-therapists may act out their own unresolved family dynamics vis-á-vis their clients and each other. There are cases in which the therapist makes a patient into his or her parent or sibling in order to seek the approval or admiration of the patient. A female therapist was particularly enamored with an older man who had come into treatment with his family. As an expert in sex therapy, she had a well-founded suspicion that impotence lay at the core of the trouble the parents had with their daughter, the identified patient. The therapist was reluctant to move the therapy in the direction it needed to go and continued to bask in the glowing approval the man directed her way: she was so competent for one so young, so intelligent and interesting. Her co-therapist did not comment on the situation because he treated her as a beloved younger sister. In his family, his sister never received the attention she wanted from her father, and he enjoyed watching his co-therapist find acceptance in the eyes of their patient. The eldest daughter in the family precipitated a crisis, the family terminated abruptly, and the mother sought a women's group to discuss her problems. They were not getting help, so they found a way to leave.

In another case, a codependent couple entered co-therapy treatment. The male therapist persisted in "rescuing" the female client, who was alcoholic. Whenever her husband or the female co-therapist would address the woman about the consequences of her behavior, the male therapist would speak on behalf of the patient. As the child of an alcoholic himself, he was aware of this tendency in himself but rationalized his behavior as necessary to keep the woman in treatment. His co-therapist was frustrated but accepted his rationale because he was the more experienced family therapist in the treatment of couples, a skill she wanted to learn from him. The co-therapy team became enmeshed in the family's system of denial. The therapy terminated when the female therapist withdrew from her co-therapy contract and offered to work with the family alone. No change was possible in the system that they had created.

A third case, involves two female co-therapists who treated a group that included a 24-year-old male who suffered from a borderline personality disorder. Both therapists were overly careful and solicitous with him as if he were extremely fragile which he was not. Both skirted the issue of his illness, although he described out of body experiences and was exceedingly enraged at both of them and the group. Although both were skilled at setting boundaries in group therapy, neither set limits on his behavior and did not support group members' efforts to do so. The group was threatened and angry at the therapists, and several members left because they felt unsafe. Neither therapist questioned the appropriateness of this group for the patient. The co-therapists acted as if they were enthralled by the patient and his manipulations. Both had come from families with schizophrenic parents, and they were deeply afraid to use their clinical acumen as they knew best. They feared he would go completely crazy, and it would be their fault. Once their belief was exposed in talks with a group therapy consultant, the co-therapy team was able to establish a group environment that isolated the borderline pathology. Seeing that he could no longer intimidate the co-therapists or the group, the patient left treatment.

Another co-therapy team, both males, failed to identify their own tendency to project onto their patients because their projection helped them "resolve" their own competitive urges and let them avoid conflict between themselves. The team unconsciously selected a convenient male target in their treatment group and projected their unwanted competitive energy onto him. Unfortunately, their collusion coincided with a general inclination by the group as a whole to scapegoat this member. Not only did the therapists confront the patient about his "excessive rivalry" but the group expressed their displeasure about his "unnecessary aggressiveness." The therapists did not protect him from the wrath of the group. The patient developed an iatrogenic condition of anxiety and fear based on his negative group experience, and he left treatment in dismay. The therapists remained blind to their complicity in the scapegoating of the patient until after the fact of his departure from the group, when the competitive behavior between them emerged strongly. They sought third-party consultation. Their difficulty stemmed from unrecognized sibling rivalry that they unwittingly acted out during group sessions. With assistance, they were able to improve their effectiveness in group, but their awareness came too late to help the scapegoated male.

Co-therapists can collude with the group as a whole in order to avoid the emergence of a particular issue in the group. An example of this was the male–female co-therapy team who disliked anger and supported their group's desire to bypass the slightest arousal of hostility. The therapists proved successful in their efforts to placate all acrimony before it flourished but complained that the group was "boring" and not very active. They sought out the help of a group consultant in order to bring some life into the group process. The consultant pointed out the discrepancy between what they wanted on a conscious level, that is, a lively and functional group, and what they acted out on an unconscious level, a profound evasion of all animosity. The group had stalled because it could not progress deeper than the co-therapists would allow. With direction from their consultant, the therapists began their first tentative experiments with permitting the expression of anger in the group. At first the group turned their suppressed feelings of anger onto the co-therapists, which fulfilled their worst fears. However, the group gradually evolved a culture that permitted the expression of an entire range of feelings and let closeness and intimacy flower among the members.

Co-therapists can also collude against the group as a whole. This condition can approach the dimensions of a paranoid delusion, especially in the case where the therapists see the group as an abusive parent or sibling. This is more likely to occur in an institutional setting where the therapists may be required to conduct a therapy group because of the clinic's needs and not their desire to lead. One such example occurred in a private psychiatric hospital whose clinical administration initiated an ill-conceived treatment plan. Two therapists were called on to conduct an inpatient group of borderline and other highly dysfunctional patients, although both therapists lacked both the training and motivation to lead this kind of specialized group. The therapists were afraid of the patients and projected onto them their own anxiety and hostility. The patients responded with abusive outbursts at their co-therapists, who began to see the group as the abusive mother and father they had entered the field of mental health to escape. The group took on an ugly mood and developed a siege mentality, each side ready to attack any vulnerability exposed by the other. The therapists retreated to the nursing station following each group, and the patients hovered about the door waiting for one of them to appear. The treatment milieu was rife with signs of paranoia. After 2 months, neither group members nor leaders showed up at the appointed hour. The plan of the hospital administration had been passively defeated, but at a high cost for those involved. The co-therapists had paired with each other against the group in an attempt to manage their own feelings of fear and anger.

Another dysfunctional model is the scapegoated co-therapist. Whenever a new therapist enters an established group, there is an opportunity to single out the new leader for persecution of some kind. If the original therapist does not welcome the presence of the new therapist for whatever reason, there is a strong tendency to exclude the new therapist from the group culture. Unfortunately, institutional settings often provide the backdrop for these dramas because therapists are sometimes coerced into doing co-therapy with people they do not choose and are then required to treat "difficult" patients. Also, therapists sometimes attempt to lead groups or conduct family therapy sessions without sufficient training and/or supervision. These pressures conspire to produce an unwholesome atmosphere for psychotherapy and co-therapy. Whenever one therapist colludes with the group or family to exclude or chastise the second therapist, an untenable therapeutic environment is created.

In the private sector, scapegoating of this kind usually replays "If it Weren't for You," a psychological game (Berne, 1964) that puts the blame on the other therapist for deficiencies in the therapy. However, it only serves temporarily to forestall the patients' anxiety about their own acceptability. Eventually, the issue of what will be tolerated must come to the forefront if therapy is going to progress. In one case, the colluding therapist was a woman who satisfied an unrecognized script of loyalty in her family of origin by siding with the group against her male co-therapist in much the same way she had sided with her mother against her father. The male co-therapist was bewildered and subsequently left the group. Co-therapists find it very nearly impossible to define the issues in this kind of countertransference because the processes are so powerful and unconscious. Third-party intervention is necessary. The experience of being scapegoated by either a family or a group is one of the most painful that a psychotherapist can endure. Many therapists never return to group or family therapy after undergoing the trauma. The fact that your co-therapist has colluded against you only adds insult to injury.

Sometimes a therapist selects a family member or group member as his or her "co-therapist" and excludes his or her actual co-therapist. This kind of pairing occurs because patients consistently offer themselves as "helpers" to one or the other therapist. A therapist who permits such a split to occur runs the risk of compromising the entire enterprise of co-therapy. The co-therapist who is being excluded will become very angry and hurt. The other patients will become quite confused and wonder, "Who are the leaders?" They may also experience envy that the therapist has chosen one person as a special "helper" over all the rest. The patient who is chosen must give up his or her needs in an effort to meet the standards of a co-therapist. A therapist who colludes with a patient in this way may be passively expressing his or her dissatisfaction or anger at his or her co-therapist. This kind of indirect maneuver will never meet the conditions of adequate co-therapy.

Another variation on the theme of excluding a co-therapist is the situation in which one therapist becomes the "trustworthy" therapist in the discussion of shared secrets and verbal intimacies. A female client called Bill on the phone to share an erotic dream and express her sexual attraction to him. She insisted that he not speak to Vivian about it. "I would be too embarassed to return to group if you did," she said. Bill replied that the rule for co-therapy was "no secrets" between co-therapists and that he had an obligation to reveal to Vivian the substance of their conversation. He pointed out the similarity between the way she tried to manipulate him and the way her father had manipulated her when he committed acts of sexual abuse with her. The patient said she was angry and that she felt rejected by Bill. The following week she returned to group and expressed relief that Bill had reinforced the boundary between them, something her father had never done. She was relieved and felt protected by the co-therapy team. The policy of "no secrets" between co-therapists has proven to be of enormous clinical significance over the years. Co-therapists who depart from this rule do so at the peril of the co-therapy treatment. Usually, they cultivate "private understandings" with patients apart from their co-therapist in order to gratify their own need to feel special in the eyes of the patient.

In Chapter 6, we elaborate on the various expressions of countertransference that co-therapists manifest in response to splitting by patients.

Any diversion of attention away from clients and onto the therapists that occurs on a regular basis becomes a disservice to the clients. Co-therapists who share a few facts about their vacation with their clients are acting appropriately. However, if they boast each week about the book they are writing or the course they are teaching, the clients are being used for therapist gratification, and the clients will justifiably resent it. Co-therapists who fight with each other during sessions over how best to proceed in the therapy fail to keep the clients at the center of the treatment process. Open disagreements with a co-therapist in the service of the clients' interests may sometimes be indicated but will distract from the clients if they become a frequent occurrence. In general, co-therapists should seek to minimize whatever takes the focus away from the clients during therapy.

When co-therapists adopt the dysfunctional family roles that they enacted in their families of origin, the treatment process falters. For example, a male–female co-therapy team was treating a substance-abusing mother, her husband, and two preadolescent children in family therapy. The mother exuded a Blanche Dubois kind of frailty during family sessions, and the male co-therapist played the "Rescuer" to her "Victim" (Karpman, 1968). He was accustomed to this role as a child, and although he had analyzed it in his own psychotherapy, he felt more comfortable in that position, especially in the beginning stages of family treatment. His female co-therapist played the "Persecutor" and, like her male counterpart, felt accustomed to this role by virtue of her own family experience. She challenged the mother whenever she passively broke her agreements with her family. The male therapist stroked her for her courage to continue treatment, and the female therapist confronted her for noncompliance. This rigid way of relating to the patient repeated in cyclic fashion across several months while the treatment languished at an impasse.

During a session with a co-therapy supervisor, the inflexibility of the co-therapy team became obvious to the therapists. They agreed to share alternately the roles of carrot and stick, although neither therapist felt comfortable doing so. The switch brought an immediate reaction from the client. She became furious at the male therapist when he confronted her because it elicited transferential feelings concerning her father. She also grieved deeply for her dead mother when the female therapist showed her caring. The transition of the therapists from their family roles produced an important shift in the therapy. As a rule of thumb, co-therapists should consciously experiment with various ways of relating to their patients, if only to avoid familiar roles that may block therapeutic progress. For example, the therapist who is the comforter and nurturer will become more questioning, and the practical-minded efficiency expert will become more attentive to intuitive clues and dream material.

### Confusion and Lack of Communication

Confusion and the absence of clarity in the communication between co-therapists and between clients and co-therapists are present to some degree in most paradigms of co-therapy dilemmas. The self, the relationship, and the task are the three dimensions that co-therapists can talk about. Failure to talk about any or all of these dimensions can lead to negative consequences as the following examples show.

Whenever therapists are not clear with each other about their understanding of their patients and their goals for the therapy, clients will become baffled, and the therapy will suffer. It is sometimes difficult for the therapists to discover how their lack of clarity produced confusion in their patients, but it is useful for co-therapists to look for clues.

For example, Bill spontaneously began speaking to a couple in co-therapy treatment about the need for them to commit to an intimate relationship. He had not consulted Vivian about this change in strategy, although they had treated the couple as patients for 2 years. The result was confusion on the part of Vivian and terror on the part of the couple, who promptly left treatment. The merits of spontaneity aside, discussion of decisions that alter the course of treatment are necessary to prepare not only co-therapists for a shift in direction but also their patients. Although the error appeared quite obvious in retrospect, it was several weeks before we both comprehended how we had slighted the co-therapy process.

Patients will be confused by the unequal status of a nequipo team if that status is implicitly denied or a proper explanation is not forthcoming. Once, a supervisor wanted to move his trainee into competency equal to himself quicker than was prudent or even realistically possible. His trainee picked up on the "Hurry up" driver and wanted to please her teacher. She was a bright student and an accomplished therapist in her own right but lacked both knowledge and experience in group psychotherapy. Both supervisor and trainee sought to ignore this significant disparity in their relationship and chose to act as if they were peers and not nequipos. They neglected to mention her status as a trainee to their psychotherapy group and led them to believe by omission that the two were equal partners. Since they were the same age and treated each other as equals, it was not difficult for the members to see them as full-fledged co-therapists. After 6 months, he took a vacation and left her in charge of the group by herself. He was confident that she could handle any crisis that occurred. Once he was gone, the group unloaded a tremendous amount of pent-up hostility on his co-therapist, thinking she could handle it. She cracked under the weight of their anger, which she had not expected and had no resources to maintain her equilibrium. It became clear to the group that she was incapable of leading them, and they left *en masse*. The supervisor returned to a trainee who never wanted to lead groups again and to clients furious because they had been deceived. The nequipos had killed their group by their neglect to disclose fully the nature of their relationship. Patients have a right to know the unequal status of their leaders.

Sometimes the lack of communication between co-therapists can reach humorous proportions. Once there was a co-therapy pair who tried to maintain equality in their relationship by alternating couple therapy appointments between their respective offices that were in different cities. The male co-therapist had much difficulty remembering not only the place of each meeting but also the day and time. His behavior produced a comedy of errors. Sometimes the couples would have unexpected solo appointments. Other times, only the first half of the therapy hour was solo because the forgetful therapist would arrive at last. Often the therapy would take place outside the locked office door of the erring therapist who traveled to the wrong office. After a while, the forgetful behavior became infectious. The couples in treatment became so confused that they began showing up at the wrong place and winding up at the right place tardy. Even the female therapist began mimicking her absent-minded partner.

Clearly, this was a disruptive pattern that confused everyone concerned. Both the clients and the female therapist had shown extraordinary flexibility, but their patience had grown thin. The male therapist was distracted by discordant events in his own life. His co-therapist was able to put up with his forgetfulness because he shared his personal distress with her, and she understood that his lapses of memory were a temporary condition. Also, she benefited because he was outstanding in the therapy itself. Together they formulated a plan whereby he would call her and check the location and time for all appointments. Although this was a highly codependent strategy, it improved the male therapist's attendance at sessions. Finally, a plan was devised whereby all participants in the therapy wrote the day, time, and place for the next appointment in little books and stated it aloud in order to synchronize their activity. A workable pattern of communication was at last established.

### Lack of Congruence between Co-Therapists

Therapists who do not perceive the patient's illness in roughly similar fashion run the risk of placing him or her in a double bind. In general, they must agree on the diagnosis and the severity of the condition of the patient or the family in order to formulate a coherent treatment plan and not sabotage each other's efforts. For example, two therapists were treating a 30-year-old male patient in group therapy. The female co-therapist chose to see grave pathology in the patient's character and gave him the diagnosis of borderline personality disorder. Her male co-leader, however, chose to view the patient's idiosyncrasies from a nonpathological model and described him as a fascinating character with imaginative though somewhat weird dreams. The therapists recognized the discrepancies but perceived themselves as flexible and mature clinicians who were above such disputes.

The treatment of the patient proceeded in orderly fashion until the patient insisted on the therapists telling him the truth and raised the following questions: "Am I sick or not?" and "How deep is my illness?" and "How long must I be in treatment?" These questions forced the co-therapists to face their disparity of opinion, which they had adroitly avoided. In order to respond directly to the patient's inquiries, the co-therapists devoted considerable time to discussing how best to define the psychotherapy treatment to the patient. Both clinicians were adequately trained in psychopathology but were unable to reach agreement on either the diagnosis or severity of illness in this man's case. They decided to present contradictory impressions to the patient. The female therapist recommended to him that he undertake individual as well as group therapy and predicted a five year course of treatment. The male therapist recommended that he continue group therapy and declined to comment on the length of treatment. In the face of such starkly disparate opinions, the patient's anxiety and confusion peaked. Within three weeks, he left therapy without notice and was hospitalized by the police for bizarre behavior. The co-therapists had placed him in a double bind, and he chose to go crazy.

Co-therapists are sometimes able to possess a wide variance of opinions and yet coordinate themselves as a co-therapy team. The patients they treat, however, are not so flexible. They may be obsessed with the questions of "Who is right?" and "What should I do?" With these questions, they seek to quell their own anxiety and make sense of their treatment. An example of this was a 45-year-old woman in family therapy whose co-therapists differed on how best to treat her depressed condition. One therapist believed medication and individual therapy were indicated in addition to family treatment. The other therapist recommended intensive family therapy and no medication or individual therapy because he did not want to support the husband's perception of his wife as the identified patient. Both co-therapists had similar theoretical backgrounds and psychotherapy training but clearly disagreed in the case of this family. They offered both options for the patient to choose. The woman chose medication with individual therapy to monitor compliance because, in her words, "I don't want to bother my wonderful family with my own petty problems." She abruptly refused to meet with the family again in therapy and thanked the medicating therapist profusely for "saving" her marriage. The co-therapists blamed each other for "losing" the family therapy. The patient succeeded in driving a wedge between the co-therapists such that they no longer wished to continue their collaboration. She did this out of her need to cope with her anxiety and her need to obtain clarity in an ambiguous situation created by the therapists. The co-therapists' incongruence provided the avenue for her to avoid her work and sabotaged their relationship in the process.

Another case of co-therapist incongruence developed when two highly skilled male therapists attempted to co-lead a group together. They liked each other personally and respected each other's achievements as healers. However, they underestimated the impact that the divergence of their theoretical beliefs would have on their patients. One therapist, Jim, treated the group-as-a-whole and made references to each individual's behavior in light of group phenomena. The other therapist, Charles, continually interrupted the group process because he treated individuals in a group setting and never focused on the phenomena of the group-as-a-whole. The group members were confounded. Some wanted to follow Jim's way and others chose Charles' strategy. A division occurred within the group, and each member had to choose between the two therapists. Those loyal to Jim were furious at Charles' interruptions and berated him whenever he began individual treatment in the group. Those partial to Charles' methods complained that Jim was not active enough. They attacked Jim's supporters and defended Charles' preference for individual treatment. Group members ceased to cooperate with each other, and they squabbled over who was right. Although the therapists were able to tolerate the wide divergence of their beliefs, the group members in treatment could not. The group's strong reaction forced the therapists to reconsider their decision to work together because the members were not being served well. They decided to split the group along theoretical lines and allow each person to join the therapist he or she wished. So ended an ill-conceived co-therapy experiment because the incompatibility of the co-therapists' theoretical beliefs was too great. No matter how much flexibility and understanding co-therapists demonstrate between themselves, they must be able to coordinate their therapeutic efforts if their patients are going to benefit from the treatment.

Frequently, therapists who are physicians and therapists who are not manifest incongruence over the medication of a patient. For example, a depressed male patient named Rupert received subliminal contradictory messages when one therapist approved and supplied antidepressant medication for him, even though the other strongly disapproved. Co-therapist incongruence, albeit not overtly expressed in treatment sessions, set the stage for acting out. Rupert was treated in a homogeneous group of depressed outpatients some of whom were medicated and some of whom were not. He began a period of non-compliance with the medical regimen prescribed for him. The co-therapist who had prescribed his medication admonished him, and the other co-therapist remained silent, tacitly supporting his acting out. Although the co-therapists had discussed between themselves their differences in the case of medicating Rupert, they neglected to see how their incongruence might affect his noncompliance. In his group, Rupert held the special leadership role of defiant leader (See Appendix, Emerging Leaders). One of his special functions in the group was to challenge the authority of the group leaders. Rupert did this on the topic of medication and succeeded in convincing other medicated persons in his group not to comply, much to the dismay of both therapists. Another of Rupert's special functions in group was to assert individual autonomy and seek a special contract with the therapists apart from his group. He did this by disparaging the usefulness of the group and requesting individual therapy with the nonmedical co-therapist. At this point, the co-therapists sought consultation. The consultant helped them see that Rupert had called into question the very existence of the group as a response to his anxiety in the face of contradictory messages by the co-therapists. The co-therapists quickly amended the situation. They acknowledged to Rupert their differences, discontinued his medica-tion, and kept him in group treatment. In the conflict described above, it is important to note that the nonmedical therapist is sometimes the one advocating medication and the medical therapist questioning its validity.

Co-therapists can also lack congruence as to the timing of termina-tion. For one year, Vivian had treated a couple with her co-therapist George. During one session, she responded positively to the man's comment that they had achieved their goals in therapy. Following the session, George confronted Vivian with the question, "Do you want to stop doing co-therapy with me?" George had taken her comment personally. He was disappointed because he believed that Vivian wanted to terminate their collaboration and not just end the couple's course of treatment. He was angry because it was clear to him that the couple had more work to do, especially with regard to intimacy. Vivian believed that the couple had reached the goals they had set for themselves at the start of therapy. She was also responding to the couple's eagerness to stop therapy, and so she supported their resis-tance to continue. Serious misunderstandings were prevented by George's confrontation. Vivian and George might have ended their co-therapy relationship, and George might have continued to treat the couple alone—angry that he had been rejected by Vivian, or the couple might never have returned to therapy under the false impression that they had completed their work. As it was, the co-therapists agreed to discuss with the couple George's ideas concerning new goals the couple could set for themselves if they decided to continue. The couple completed two more years of treatment and accomplished much more than they had thought possible. Since termination is an event fraught with many emotions for both therapists and clients, co-therapists must agree to discuss how and when it will be accomplished.

### Co-Dependency between Co-Therapists

Whereas most of our respondents agreed that reliance on a co-therapist was desirable, the specter of being dependent on one was not. Most persons want a co-therapist with whom they can learn and develop, but a few select a co-therapist in order to avoid growth.

For example, an experienced and successful male psychotherapist named Henry always chose a younger female co-therapist whenever he formed a group. He had never led a group by himself and let the presence of his co-leader assuage his fears of becoming an autonomous group therapist. His fears were so great that when his co-leader was ill or absent, he would cancel the group entirely, a practice that the group members greatly resented. He was active in group but showed undue deference to his female therapist, which, although flattering at first, became grating to her over time. She resented his dependence and expressed dissatisfaction to him that she had to shun innovative experiments in the group because she could not trust him to be there as a support. For example, when she confronted group members, he did not complement her efforts by asking them their feelings about what she was saying. Once the group ended, his co-therapist did not choose to work with him again. Determined to conquer his fears, he began once more with a new group and a new female co-therapist and again repeated the cycle. Consequently, he never developed a mature co-therapy relationship but always remained in the shadow of his partner.

This is a case of an unacknowledged nequipo (non-equal) team that poses as a co-therapy team for the treatment group. Henry employed therapists as if he were their equal, and when his inequality was exposed in group, they left his employment. In order to transcend his cycle of dependency, Henry must design a nequipo learning contract with a therapist that allows him to develop as a group leader. Although Henry is the more experienced therapist, under such a contract, Henry would be considered the assistant therapist, and his younger employee would be the therapist because of her proficiency in group treatment. Solo leadership of a group should also be required as a part of his development. Nequipo learning contracts should always address the issue of dependency and spell out as clearly as possible the responsibilities that the assistant therapist is expected to assume. The assistant therapist will sabotage the contract if he or she sits back and lets the other do the work. In nequipo teams, the trainees may be tempted to be dependent and overcompliant, especially if the therapist is a supervisor and in a position to grade them for a class or evaluate them for hours of experience. The nequipo learning contract must take this into account.

Dependency can be manifest in more subtle ways. A person can collude with his or her co-therapist so that no sensitive points will ever be revealed in their talks following sessions. For example, the female therapist who worked with Henry might have perpetuated the co-dependency simply by avoiding mention of his dependency. She might

have been tempted to continue their co-dependency if she were capti-
vated by his prestige or the number of referrals he generated and
wanted to keep her job with him.

Another example is the therapist who denies destructive behavior in
his co-therapist. A 30-year-old social worker enjoyed doing family
therapy with a 35-year-old psychiatrist, but he noticed signs of irrita-
bility and hypersensitivity in her movements and expressions. Since he
was knowledgeable in the area of substance abuse, he suspected that
she might be addicted. When she joked about her marijuana use and
how it affected her contact lenses, his suspicions were confirmed, but
he made no effort to inquire further. He did not want to know more
because he was afraid it might jeopardize a stimulating co-therapy
relationship. The psychiatrist continued to show addictive signs and
carried numerous prescription drugs in the pockets of her coat, drugs
that she displayed before her co-therapist from time to time. Still, he
did not confront. One day, she failed to show for their group session
and gave no call. She had been stopped for a traffic violation, found to
be under the influence of drugs, and ordered to a detoxification program. The group ended soon after, and the collaboration between the
therapists never resumed.

Co-therapists can also ignore their partner's countertransference,
narcissism, or other personality traits even when these pose a hazard to
the therapy itself. For example, a female therapist refused to challenge
her male co-therapist when he seductively stared at a patient's breasts
and legs in family therapy. The patient was a sexually acting-out
16-year-old who was brought into treatment by her parents in order to
prevent her from "becoming a bad influence on the younger children."
The therapist admitted to his co-therapist that the girl reminded him of
his younger sister when she was a teenager and recognized that countertransference might be a problem. He was so genuine and sincere in
his expression that his co-therapist did not want to embarrass him by
pointing out his lascivious gazes. Finally, the 14-year-old sister in the
family broke the silence and confronted the male therapist by saying,
"You look at Tina just like Dad does sometimes." The therapist was
mortified and left the session. He later asked his co-therapist to treat
the family by herself. She did so and colluded again to help him avoid
analyzing his own seductive responses.

Co-learners (non-therapist co-leaders) often demonstrate a tendency to hide behind each other so that neither takes responsibility for
the group. Supervisors contracted to train co-learners must be cognizant of this fact and encourage risk taking and autonomous action by
their trainees. A "Be perfect" driver (Kahler & Capers, 1974) may
paralyze both co-learners because it does not permit any action except

the "perfect" one. Bill once supervised a co-learner team frozen by such a dilemma. Both co-learners had the strategy of "watch for the mistakes of your partner." They became critical judges of each other, and the therapy did not progress. Employing paradoxical intent, he instructed each student consciously to make one common error in group therapy each week. The prescribed errors included calling a patient by the wrong name or forgetting some important event that had happened the week before. The co-learners so much enjoyed each others' attempts to make mistakes that they laughed openly in the group. The spell of perfection was broken.

Unfortunately, performance anxiety and the fear of exposing one's limitations as a therapist to a colleague are not confined to co-learners. Experienced therapists often are reluctant to show less than out-standing ability. Ironically, this fear may increase with the skill and expertise of the professional. As one well-known clinician put it, "I have to hit a home run each time I'm up at bat." To work under such impossible performance standards puts intolerable pressure on a co-therapy team and is, in fact, an inadequate model for patients who are always relieved and gratified when therapists do make mistakes. Co-therapists should expect competence from each other, not perfection.

A co-therapy team is heading for trouble whenever one therapist is not permitted to be equal with the other. For example, a male psychi-atrist and a female marriage and family therapist implicitly agreed not to be equal in any sense in order to keep the power on the side of the doctor and the deference on the side of the marriage and family therapist. This arrangement was lucrative for the marriage and family therapist, and the psychiatrist was comfortable not having his authority questioned. However, their tacit understanding engendered many problems for the families they treated. In particular, women trying to individuate in their families did not feel supported and couples attempting to balance the power in their own relationships were confused and disheartened by the inequality portrayed by their family therapists. Male superiority is a societal imprint for most clients in treatment, and this assumption was not called into question by either co-therapist. Instead, both reinforced the belief by modeling inequal-ity, and they remained seemingly oblivious to the quandary they created for their patients. Such co-therapy teams are especially offen-sive to women clients, as evidenced by the example Mary Goulding gives in Chapter 8 (p. 200). Unequal co-therapy contracts can lead to acting out and destructive behavior on the part of clients as Virginia Satir describes in Chapter 9 (p. 217).

It is a distortion of the co-therapy contract if either therapist requires or permits the dependency of a partner. Many of these problems can be anticipated and prevented if a proper co-therapy contract is established. The question of codependence cuts to the heart of the co-therapy enterprise. Co-therapists must be autonomous and yet must engage in a cooperative effort to heal patients. How cooperation and autonomy are balanced is the true art of co-therapy.

## SPECIAL PROBLEMS AND VULNERABILITY OF LOVERS AND MARRIAGE PARTNERS WHO ENTER INTO CO-THERAPY RELATIONSHIPS

The bonds of conjugal and otherwise openly committed couples are especially vulnerable in several ways and, in particular, to the threat of unrecognized competition. An outstanding male therapist, Phillip, and his wife of twenty years, Madeleine, decided to begin collaboration as co-therapists. Madeleine had begun the study of psychology a year earlier and desired to be a therapist herself. Phillip was a well-known psychodramatist and invited Madeleine to join him in his groups. They began work as a typical nequipo team, Madeleine eager to learn and Phillip encouraging her development. However, within a year Madeleine had demonstrated a flair for psychodrama and not only equaled Phillip but exceeded him in her facility with group. Phillip was inwardly shaken, though outwardly he remained composed. He began to criticize Madeleine, at first in a subtle way but gradually increasing in harshness and severity. Madeleine did not understand the shift in his demeanor toward her but continued to grow in her proficiency in the field. Eventually Phillip found an excuse not to work with Madeleine and suggested that she leave the field entirely because in his words she did not "possess the cognitive grasp of group process." Madeleine did not believe this and sought out supervision for her work as a therapist. The relationship between the couple had deteriorated slowly and was beginning to show signs of strain. Madeleine confronted Phillip with her suspicion that he was jealous of her ability and angry that she had dared compete with him in his own area of expertise. As Madeleine developed professionally, Phillip grew more distant and finally asked for a divorce. All of this had occurred within three years' time. The couple attempted therapy, but it was clear from the start there was no good faith on Phillip's part to maintain their union. Madeleine had moved beyond her husband's narcissistic shadow, and Phillip could not tolerate the change.

The story of Phillip and Madeleine portrays the dark side of the fond wish that many couples have to work together. In the process of collaboration, competitive urges arise where they had not been before and startle couples with their primitive force. Not all couples can manage the powerful emotions that can emerge once the collaborative process has begun. The wise couple will assess these dangers before they embark on a course of co-therapy. Co-therapy may be a hazard to the health of a relationship. Mary Goulding provides another example of this hazard in Chapter 8 (p. 200). We provide some guidelines below for couples seeking to prevent the dissolution of their bonds. These are questions couples should ask before they undertake co-therapy.

Besides professional competition, partners can be jealous of a client's attraction to their spouse. This can be manifest in the partner's reaction to the client's transference and especially transferential dreams that carry an erotic power. For example, Luisa co-led a therapy group with her husband, Brendan. A very attractive female client transferred the powerful erotic feelings she experienced for her father to Brendan, and these feelings appeared graphically in the dreams she revealed to the group. In the dreams, she and Brendan were attached sexually, and the emotional intensity she displayed as she spoke of the dreams was impossible to disguise. Luisa was disturbed by the erotic nature of the client's transference and, following group sessions, castigated Brendan for inviting the dreams. Although both therapists knew how disturbed the client was, both reacted to the patient's dreams as if they were overtures by an impetuous lover. Brendan was pleased by them and saw in them a deepening of the client's transference. Luisa was shocked by Brendan's reaction and angry that he would find pleasure in such "disgusting" images. The couple sought marital therapy in order to reduce the tension in their relationship. Luisa discovered that she could not tolerate the sexual advances of a client toward her husband and left the co-therapy team to work as a therapist on her own and in collaboration with another male therapist. In the absence of Luisa, Brendan discovered that he needed the presence of a female therapist in order to establish a boundary between himself and seductive clients. The couple discovered they could not work as a married team in the highly charged atmosphere of co-therapy, and they found other partners with whom they could work.

A co-therapist can also fall in love with his or her patient. This is a particularly painful experience for the partner since he or she not only loses the affection of husband or wife but also loses the relationship with the patient. Ginger, a vibrant therapist of 40, became enamored with a distinguished male client whom she was treating with her husband, Fred. She began to have dreams of the client, which at first she shared with Fred. As the dreams became more intense and erotic in nature, she became more reticent to tell them to her husband. Fred asked if she had ceased to dream of the client, and she was silent. Her silence aroused Fred's suspicion, which in time grew to a jealous passion. He accused her of harboring erotic wishes for their client, an accusation she could not deny because she did have waking fantasies concerning him. Fred grew cold and distant with the client and considered referring him to another co-therapy team for individual treatment. Ginger chose to return to individual therapy to confront her uncontrolled fascination for their client. Her psychotherapist encouraged her to develop boundaries between herself and the client. In order to do this, she discovered that her relationship with her husband had to change as well. Her idealization of their marriage crumbled, and in its place she constructed a picture that reflected more realistically the practical basis for their union. She realized that she had to give up her little girl fantasies that she projected onto their client as the perfect father who could satisfy her wishes. Once Ginger established emotional boundaries between herself and the client, Fred was able to relinquish his fits of jealousy and relate to Ginger as a loving husband.

Work as a co-therapy team can suddenly and surprisingly expose the inequality that exists in a marriage relationship. Bud and Wendy were marriage and family therapists who shared a private practice and treated several couples in co-therapy. Bud prided himself in his liberal beliefs toward women, and he considered himself a feminist. In fact, he was adept at helping males see their own prejudicial attitudes about women and the degree to which that affected their relationship with their wives and daughters. However, when decisions about the co-therapy needed to be made, Bud exerted considerable control and usually insisted that his way be followed. Wendy appeased Bud's desire to be in control although she resented her submission and was angry at herself when she gave in. Wendy adapted to this situation until her peer consultation group indicated how damaging her obedience could be to the couples they were treating. Wendy confronted Bud and demanded that he share the decision-making power with her. Bud was shocked and hurt because he did not want to see the part of himself that subscribed to inequality between husband and wife. His new awareness profoundly affected their marriage and the parenting of their children that had largely been under his command. Bud saw Wendy as an extension of himself and could not imagine how she might have an idea that differed from his. He had been able to sustain this idea in his marriage, but the co-therapy relationship forced him to see he was mistaken.

Vivian and Bill have experienced session spillover from co-therapy with couples in crisis. Several times we began fighting spontaneously at the close of a session, mimicking the exact conflict of the couple with whom we had just completed therapy. The content of the altercation is never the point but the process we repeat is identical to the clients' process. Bill usually sees the pattern first. As soon as one of us "calls the game," the fight ends. It is very difficult to identify and stop an altercation of this kind. Couples who do not recognize this mimicking behavior could believe incorrectly that the fight belongs to them and requires resolution. Some couples do not fight but experience a mood change following a treatment session. Couples who practice co-therapy must know their own psychological games so that they can distinguish between their own unresolved issues and those of the couples they treat.

Some couples enter into co-therapy contracts to treat couples *in order to solve* their own relationship issues. Golden and Golden warn of this occurrence among sex therapists:

> Married therapists whose sexual relationships still contain significant problems may become sex therapists as an effort, probably unconscious, to resolve the problems. They will probably run into the same impasses and blind spots as any individual who is drawn to the field of psychotherapy as a means of resolving personal problems." (Golden & Golden, 1976, p. 11)

Attempts to address marital problems by treating couples in distress is always misguided and leads to co-therapy dysfunction. We advise that co-therapy couples have their own therapy as a means to prevent co-therapy breakdown. Personal therapy is a comfort and support to co-therapists who do work at this intimate and intense level.

We want to include a precautionary note for non-therapist spouses who may feel justifiably excluded from the intimate circle that the co-therapy team creates for itself. The special nature of the co-therapy relationship and its demands on their mates' time can provoke jealousy in the most trusting and well-adjusted spouses. The establishment of a co-therapy team should not threaten the spouses of the co-therapists. If it does, we recommend that therapists and their spouses seek therapy for themselves. Some therapists may have to choose their marriages over their co-therapy.

## GUIDELINES FOR CO-THERAPY COUPLES

The following are questions a couple should consider before embarking on collaboration as co-therapists. They should discuss these from time to time as part of the on-going dialogue that partners need to keep abreast of changes in each other and the relationship.

1. What is our chief motive for being together as a couple?
2. What is our chief motive for working together?
3. Do I know what my partner wants as a result of our collaboration? Am I clear about what I want?
4. What is my greatest fear about sharing work with my partner? What is my fear if I do not work with my partner?
5. What will I want to avoid most in our work together?
6. What is my degree of commitment to our personal relationship? Can I imagine how it might be threatened by our working together?
7. How much time per week am I willing to devote to our collaboration?
8. What do I need to feel secure in my relationship? What can my partner do to enhance my sense of security?
9. How long do I want the work contract to be? Experimental time frame of _____ months? Strictly time limited? Indefinite?
10. Whom would I prefer as third party consultant if we need help?

## SECRET SEXUAL INVOLVEMENT OF CO-THERAPISTS

As we mentioned in Chapter 1, there is a great temptation for co-therapists to become sexual with each other. We do not consider sexual relations between unmarried co-therapists unethical, though this behavior may be considered taboo in some communities. Co-therapists may become sexually involved as a result of their collaboration and, in some cases, may become committed partners for life. Some of these couples may choose not to reveal their sexual liaison out of personal discretion and with no clandestine purpose in mind. They are able to focus their energies on their clients and do not allow their trysts to interfere with the treatment process.

However, co-therapists who feel compelled to keep their sexual entanglement secret because of their marital status, their position in the community, or their employment within an organization are courting trouble and probably acting-out some unresolved conflicts within themselves. In these cases, the sexual activity between co-therapists may be a form of sexual acting-out that switches the focus away from the treatment of patients and onto the primary gratification of the therapists. Co-therapists are especially prone to this kind of acting-out because of the intimacy that the co-therapy relationship fosters. The therapists are stimulated to act out their feelings of intimacy rather than discuss these feelings. As Eleanore White has observed, the heightened sexual awareness between co-therapists makes them highly susceptible

(White, 1986). Our examples concern heterosexual therapists, but the caveats apply to homosexual therapists as well.

Sharon and Todd were psychologists who began their sexual activity shortly after entering a co-therapy contract to lead a borderline group. Both were young, attractive, ambitious people, eager to earn their reputation as clinicians in private practice. Though single and uncommitted to others, they chose to keep their sexual liaison secret in order to quell rumors in the professional community. Both therapists were unsure of themselves. Sharon, in particular, wished to hide her insecurity from Todd in an effort to appear mature and desirable in his eyes. When Todd began responding to the seductive statements of an attractive woman in the group, Sharon did not confront Todd. Rather, she attacked the patient for her drug use under the guise of therapeutic confrontation. In this way, she repeated her unresolved Oedipal issue because, in her family of origin, she had attacked Mother in order to gain Father's attention. Todd was startled by Sharon's attack but did not protect the patient or even comment on it in post-session discussion. He, too, was infatuated and wanted to preserve his image as a nice guy. Their silence regarding their sexual relationship penetrated their co-therapy relationship and prevented discussion of Sharon's countertransference and other mistakes the couple made. Their collusion of silence precluded outside consultation. The co-therapy was effectively undermined.

As in the case of Sharon, a co-therapist in secret liaison becomes less able to share him- or herself and more guarded in the presence of his or her lover. The willingness to keep each other fully informed is in doubt, since most lovers during the infatuation period want to express only positive comments.

If Todd and Sharon were working in an institutional setting, they might have run the risk of dismissal from work. Sex with a co-therapist comes under the general heading of sex with a co-worker. In businesses and organizations, sexual involvement between employees is viewed as a productivity problem. Two-thirds of the time supervisors will ignore sexual involvement between employees when it comes to their attention. However, when supervisors take disciplinary measures, the female is more likely to be dismissed than the male.

Many times, differences in social class and professional status are means by which one partner exercises power over the other. For example, in a large mental health clinic, a highly respected male psychiatrist took a younger female psychiatric nurse under his wing as his protege. He was married, and she was single. They had worked together in the clinic for over a year before the psychiatrist invited her to join him as co-leader in his adolescent group. They functioned as an advanced nequipo team. He admired her therapeutic assertiveness, and she respected his clinical acumen. Within the first three months, their post-session discussions expanded to include lunches and occasional after-hours meetings over coffee. They grew quite fond of each other and expressed openly their mutual sexual attraction. The professional boundaries were violated during an extended post-group session in the psychiatrist's office. She complained of tension in her neck and he responded by sitting next to her on the couch and massaging her. They became sexually intimate and began a pattern of sexual liaisons in his office after each group.

As a result of their involvement, they became less available to their adolescent patients. They became more interested in seeing each other than in seeing progress in their patients. Both were distracted from their duties by the need to protect the secrecy of their affair. Neither wished to jeopardize their positions in the clinic. Their desire to be with each other increased, as did the frequency of their sexual contact during work hours. They became more careless in their precautions and once, following group, were discovered caressing by a colleague preparing for another group. A rumor spread throughout the clinic and reached the ears of the clinic manager, who in turn confronted the psychiatrist. To assuage his feelings of guilt, the psychiatrist confessed his indiscretions and pleaded with the manager not to make public his misbehavior. The manager agreed, and the psychiatrist, as chief of the clinic, took measures to dismiss his protege and lover. She was angered and humiliated by the suggestion that she leave her job, but she complied with his wishes in order to receive excellent recommendations and his good will in the mental health establishment of their community.

A secret sexual liaison can create havoc in therapists' personal lives. Hal and Joyce were social workers in private practice in a medium-sized town in the middle West. Both were married to nontherapists, and their families were friendly. They had known each other as students in graduate school and had been colleagues for fifteen years. Joyce decided to form a family practice clinic with a pediatrician and a psychologist, and she invited Hal to join her in the business venture as her co-partner. Hal was eager to expand his practice and looked forward to a closer association with Joyce whose business sense he had always admired.

As co-directors, the pair began working 60-hour weeks developing their clinic, much of that time in intense planning and organizing between themselves. Although away from their homes most evenings, their families understood the special effort needed to start a business. They began their co-therapy career treating a co-dependent couple in family therapy. The family was difficult to treat because of their

entrenched patterns of denial and enmeshment. Following a particularly intense family session, Hal invited Joyce to have a drink with him.
His family was away on a vacation that he himself was too busy to
enjoy. He asked Joyce to come home with him that evening because he
was lonely. Joyce was surprised but also flattered because she had
always found Hal attractive. She called her husband and told him she
would be working late and went home with Hal.

Once their affair began, their hours spent together and away from
home increased. Their families became irritated, and domestic conflict
erupted. As tensions grew at home, Hal and Joyce found solace in each
other's company. Their need to maintain secrecy from their spouses as
well as their colleagues increased their co-dependency as a couple. They
established a pattern of lying and denying in the face of their spouses'
suspicions. The family they were treating noticed changes in their behavior, and the wife asked at one point if they were "burning the candle
at both ends." The co-therapists brushed aside their patient's intuitive
insight and implicitly instructed her to deny what she saw.

Hal and Joyce fused as a co-therapy unit and reinforced the co-
dependency of the family in treatment. Hal's son and Joyce's daughter
began to develop psychological symptoms that they as parents denied.
Hal gained weight and began drinking more. Joyce's husband requested marital counseling that she refused because it was, in her
words, "not my problem." Marital discord in both families had developed into full-blown crises. At last, colleagues in the family practice
clinic were able to break through their co-directors' denial by com-
plaining that the clinic was losing money. After more than a year of
subterfuge and rising hostility, Hal and Joyce attempted to mend
family ties but found they had been irreparably damaged.

Co-therapists who become involved sexually as a result of their
collaboration must understand that their involvement most likely will
produce consequences for co-therapy treatment. These consequences
may be disguised by the patients, or the co-therapists may choose not
to see the consequences because of either conscious or unconscious
motives. In each case, the co-therapists must make some decisions.
First, are they willing to reveal their liaison? If there are compelling
reasons not to reveal, are they willing to seek third-party consultation?
If they cannot agree to seek consultation, they ought to consider
terminating either the co-therapy relationship or the sexual relationship.

We have been able to help many co-therapy teams by the knowledge
we provide here. Many co-therapists who have gone off course can

restore or attain their therapeutic effectiveness and become both astute and adept in the application of their art. The prerequisite for this kind of change is awareness of the problem as it develops and willingness to confront one's partner. Such action takes courage and assertiveness, but the benefits to be gained are well worth the risks.

# ◆ 6 ◆

# *Treatment of a Borderline and a Narcissistic Patient in Co-Therapy*

This chapter describes our co-therapy treatment of two patients, each of whom is being treated in both group and individual modes. These patients have progressed moderately well and are still in psychotherapy with us at the time of this writing (1990). We report on their progress from the time they entered treatment with us until the beginning of 1989. They have been together in the same psychotherapy group since 1987. One, Kevin, a 42-year-old male, has a narcissistic personality disorder, and the other, Christine, a 34-year-old female, has a high-functioning borderline personality disorder. We analyze each patient's case with an eye to understanding specifically how co-therapy was helpful in elucidating each patient's individual psychodynamics and attenuating the psychopathology. We also discuss the specific skills co-therapists must bring to the treatment of these patients and the mistakes we made in the co-therapy.

In our survey of psychotherapists, we discovered that they preferred group therapy as the mode of treatment in which to do co-therapy. Eighty-four percent of our sample did co-therapy in group therapy, and over 50% of our sample did co-therapy in family or couple work. However, 11 therapists, almost 9% of our sample, practiced co-therapy in the individual mode. There is a small but significant number of patients who are treated by co-therapy in both the group and individual mode. We report on one such patient, Christine, in this chapter.

We focus on three topics: why co-therapy was deemed necessary as part of the treatment plan, the specific treatment options it opened up for the therapy, and the psychodynamic processes that can be worked through in the presence of a co-therapist. We discuss in detail two treatment options, reparenting and dual transference, and the co-therapy resolution of splitting, projective identification, and counter-transference.


## DIAGNOSTIC CRITERIA

Making the differential diagnosis between borderline and narcissistic personality disorders carries important implications for treatment. Therefore, we shall compare briefly the characteristics between the narcissistic person and the borderline person described in this chapter (American Psychiatric Association, 1980; Kernberg, 1975, 1980; & Masterson, 1976, 1981). Both are long-term patients with treatment over a number of years: Christine, the borderline personality, three and one-half years and still in progress; Kevin, the narcissistic personality, nine years with a hiatus of three years with no treatment and still in progress. They have committed a considerable amount of time and money toward their treatment. Both have been treated in co-therapy during a significant part of their course of psychotherapy. The characteristics that follow define these two patients.

Whereas both personalities tend to vacillate between the idealization and devaluation of important persons in their lives, and whereas both experience rage and emptiness as symptoms of their illness, there exist many significant differences in how these people behave and how they are perceived.

The narcissistic patient identifies with his mother and seeks her out for both financial and emotional supplies. He has a fused self and mother representation and assumes the characteristics of his parent. The borderline patient severely restricts contact with her mother because she experiences her mother as destructive and knows at some level that her mother has contributed to her illness. She is not fused with her parent but rather split off so that the mother is experienced as an alien and controlling force.

The narcissist has a grandiose self-representation that is fused with the omnipotent parent representation. The fusion of the self with the idealized self is a defense against rage, shame, and feelings of devaluation. The borderline, however, has not fused the self and parent representation but split them into separate rewarding and withdrawing units, which alternate repeatedly in her relationships with others. She can either cling or distance, both of which are defensive maneuvers.

Whereas the narcissist is often oblivious to his surroundings and the reactions of others, the borderline is hypersensitive to both.

The narcissist may appear invulnerable, but below the surface of the grandiosity and exaggeration is a subtle fragility. In contrast, the borderline in the clinging state appears quite fragile and yet demonstrates a cunning strength beneath the surface.

The narcissist demonstrates an overinvestment in the self by the way he is preoccupied with fantasies of unlimited success, power, brilliance, and beauty. The borderline expresses inadequacy about herself.

The narcissist knows he exists as a person, whereas the borderline experiences a severe identity disturbance concerning self-image, body image, and gender identity. The narcissist wants a mirroring of imagined perfection, whereas the borderline simply wants to know she exists, although she does seek perfection as well. The constancy of the loved person is most critical for the borderline.

The rage of the narcissist is cold and rejecting. The rage of the borderline is hot and murderous.

The narcissist envies the gifts and advantages of others and, although constantly seeking strokes, he has difficulty internalizing them when received. He also has difficulty giving strokes. The borderline has difficulty accepting strokes but gives them with greater ease.

The patients' dreams differ considerably. The dreams of the narcissist do not possess stark, primitive images. The access to primary process is not readily available. There are no obvious boundary deficiencies, no auditory or visual hallucinations, no dissociation from one's body. The dreams of the borderline often are replete with primitive symbols with a lurid, surreal, and sinister aspect to them. She experiences profound boundary deficiencies with respect to time and space. Temporally, she often experiences a memory as if it is occurring in the here and now. Spatially, she often needs greater physical distance between the therapist and herself in order to maintain a sense of her own integrity and avoid ego disintegration. She reports dissociating from her body and having out-of-body phenomena of one sort or another. Transient psychotic experiences are not uncommon, including auditory hallucinations. She experiences voices inside her head. Like many other borderlines, she often demonstrates so-called psychic abilities. In contrast with the narcissist, she possesses a high degree of empathy for others.

As to strategies of intervention, in general, we must interpret and mirror empathically the behavior of the narcissistic personality. In this manner the therapist can point out the ways in which the patient is denying, avoiding, or devaluing what is real. Confrontation too early in the treatment only served to increase his resistance and harden his false, invulnerable exterior. However, the resistance of the borderline is expressed by either withdrawal or clinging. Both are variations of acting–out and must be confronted in order to treat the underlying depression, rage, and pain. Interpretation by itself only serves to move the borderline patient into intellectualization that impedes the patient's progress in treatment. The borderline usually responds well to confrontation of her splitting. Following confrontation she is able to hear the interpretation. Her ego can integrate that information, and her immediate functioning will generally improve.

## TREATMENT OPTIONS UNIQUE TO CO-THERAPY

In our discussion of Christine and Kevin, we elaborate by examples the following treatment options that are unique to co-therapy:

*Dual transference.* Co-therapy allows the possibility of simultaneous libidinal transference to two therapists. This is problematic for borderlines and narcissists, who have difficulty in making one relationship. Both therapists must establish a therapeutic alliance with the patient. A male–female team is able to work simultaneously on gender–related issues such as trust, abuse, and sexual identity.

*Reparenting* (Schiff, 1969). This treatment strategy necessarily involves a male–female team when it seeks to replicate the primal triad. Once that is established, the patient can receive new parenting messages and corrective emotional experiences in a relationship with two parental figures. The patient must consent to the strategy of reparenting and must make an explicit contract with the therapists to do so. Most patients we treat in co–therapy do not have reparenting contracts. However, both patients in this chapter have established reparenting contracts.

## PSYCHODYNAMIC PROCESSES WORKED THROUGH BY CO-THERAPISTS

*Becoming aware of countertransference and working through in the company of a co-therapist.* Countertransference is the therapist's emotional or be havioral response to the words and actions of the patient that disturb and activate the underlying conflicts of the therapist. It becomes problematic when it goes unrecognized and unanalyzed.

*Becoming aware of projective identification and processing it in the company of a co-therapist.* In projective identification, the patient projects split off parts of the self into the therapist who then experiences being possessed by and controlled by these qualities.* Because the therapist modifies these projected parts, they are able to be reintrojected by the patient in more tolerable and less threatening forms.† This is a complicated human interaction and difficult to understand and detect when it is happening.

*Becoming aware of splitting and working through in the company of a co-therapist.* In the context of co-therapy, splitting occurs when the patient splits the co-therapy team into good and bad parts. Another variation on this theme is the fusion of the co-therapy team and then splitting between the team and the group. Sometimes one member of the co-therapy team is fused with the group and the patient splits between them and the other co-therapist. All these operations are primitive defenses of the ego.

---

*Kernberg (1980, p.27): "Projective identification, in contrast to projection, consists of the projection into another person of split-off parts of the ego or self or of an internal object. Rather than simply dissociating itself from that projected part, the ego, under the effects of projective identification, aims to forcefully enter into the external object and control it."

†Grinberg, Sor, and de Bianchedi (1977, p. 29) describe Bion's notion of projective identification as follows: ". . . parts of the ego are projected into the object, causing this object to be experienced as controlled by the projected parts and imbued with their qualities. This mechanism, active from the beginning of life, may have various functions: of relieving the ego of bad parts; of preserving good parts by protecting them from a bad internal world; of attacking and destroying the object; etc. One of the consequences of this process is that by projecting the bad parts (including fantasies and bad feelings) into a good breast (an understanding object), the infant will be able—insofar as his development allows—to reintroject the same parts in a more tolerable form, once they have been modified by the thought (reverie) of the object . . ."

Ogden (1979, p. 370): "I find Winnicott's view to be the most useful in clarifying the role of the therapist's feelings in the successful handling of a patient's projective identifications. As an object of the patient's projective identification, it is the task of the therapist both to experience and process the feelings involved in the projection. The therapist allows himself to participate to an extent in an object relationship that the patient has constructed on the basis of an earlier relationship. In so doing, the therapist has the opportunity to observe the qualities of the previously internalized object relationship and, over time, process the feelings involved in such a way that the patient is not merely repeating an old relationship in the therapy."

## CHRISTINE

> . . . often a patient relates to one therapist with relative consistency, perceiving him with minimal distortion, while working through a series of vehement, irrational, and often dramatic transference reactions to the other therapist. It appears that one therapist can be selected to represent the reality principle, allowing the patient to give fantasy reactions free play with the other therapist. A stable relationship with one therapist seems to provide a framework, or a safe anchorage, permitting the patient to feel and explore violent reactions which under other circumstances might be restrained through fear of a complete break with reality. (Mintz, 1963, pp. 127–132)

This quote is particularly pertinent to the treatment of borderlines in co-therapy. We shall illustrate the truth of Elizabeth Mintz' statement in our discussion of Christine. With this patient we have used co-therapy to provide protection for a person both emotionally and sexually abused as a child. The first year in treatment Vivian protected Christine from her memories of a sexually abusive stepfather, memories she projected onto Bill. During this time Christine experienced Bill as a bossy person who wanted to control her. By the third year of treatment, the former negative transference having been resolved to a large degree, Bill protected Christine from her memories of a neglectful, unprotective, and cold mother, memories she projected onto Vivian. Approaching three and one-half years of treatment, this is just beginning to be resolved.

The picture is even more complicated. Toward the middle and end of the second year of treatment, Christine began splitting between the two therapists, making Bill the "bad" mother and Vivian the "good" mother. The issue over which the split arose was the suitability of a certain man friend in Christine's life. Bill's tendency to be overprotective, an expression of his countertransference, was counterbalanced by Vivian's willingness to trust Christine's judgment in her choice of men and the timing of her relationships.

"It helps to have Vivian," said Christine. "It's like going to Mother, the one I never had."

Later, on the phone with Bill, afraid that she was losing him by her choice of Vivian, Christine says, "You know that I still love you." This was the first mention of love by the patient in the treatment. Then the patient described in detail how she saw herself benefiting from the co-therapy.

"I like the differences between you. I like Bill's intensity and Vivian's permissiveness. It gives me a choice. I don't have to be so dependent on Bill. I have someone else to listen to."

Our therapy began with Christine in September 1985, when she requested group psychotherapy. The group appropriate for her was one co-led by Vivian and Bill. Thus, co-therapy was introduced from the start of the treatment. Initially, she complained that she drank alcohol until unconscious on some occasions and developed only destructive and abusive relationships with men. In January 1986, the patient requested an individual session with Bill. He believed the patient would benefit from the dual transference of co-therapy in the individual mode and suggested that Vivian attend the session also. As co-therapists, we embarked on this plan because we believed it would facilitate the patient's ability to receive healthy messages about relationships between males and females. In addition, we hoped to begin a reparenting contract with the patient so that she could receive emotional nurturing. This kind of nurturing did not happen for her in the on-going group therapy because, in her own words, "The group has too many males." In fact, there were more males than females in her group.

The co-therapy did not accomplish what we intended at the time because memories of sexual abuse began to flood the patient's consciousness with such intensity that she could not remain in the same room with both therapists. The negative transference became too great for the patient to tolerate. The patient stated, "Bill is abusing me and Vivian is not protecting me." This theme has reappeared again and again across the course of treatment at varying levels of intensity. In retrospect, a form of projective identification had already begun to occur. Christine was experiencing psychotic symptoms including the loss of her body boundary and the loss of the boundary between the present and the past. As a defense, she projected her need for control into Bill, who responded by being controlling. The patient experienced his directiveness as abusive. Furthermore, she projected her neglectful mother into Vivian who remained silent and condoned Bill's behavior. We describe on page 142 below a typical interaction of this kind in the vignette, "An Example of Projective Identification."

We had expected Christine to regress but had not expected her regression to be so primitive. Luthman and Kirschenbaum (1974, p. 203) have observed a similar regressive tendency in individuals whom they treat in co-therapy. They conclude:

> . . . the co-therapy team makes it possible for the client to achieve a regressive state, sometimes instantaneously—always within a matter of three or four sessions. There is a direct parental transference which triggers early infantile conflicts. Now, we don't think that just has to do with having two therapists in the room who happen to be male and female. We think that regressive process is set off by the power of

the connection between the male and female co-therapists. If they have a connection which is discrepant with the client's original parental connection in a positive sense, then the client will often open readily, almost in spite of himself.

In March 1986, the patient terminated co-therapy in the individual mode and began a course of individual treatment with Bill alone. Psychodynamically she had recapitulated her family experience. She could not tolerate being alone with Stepfather and Mother because Stepfather would abuse her and Mother would not protect her. Yet, she trusted males more than females, who like Mother, could not be trusted. It is significant to note that in seven years of individual and group treatment prior to her experience with us, the content of sexual abuse had never entered her consciousness.

We have noted that often, as in the case of Christine, the male–female co-therapy team is better able than the solo therapist to diagnose the existence of sexual abuse in the family history of patients. This is because unconscious memories and abuse dreams emerge when the male–female dyad is presented as a treatment condition for the patient. It becomes a challenge for the co-therapists to keep a patient in treatment when this occurs. The patient will want to leave treatment in order to avoid the pain and reinforce the denial. The patient may accuse the therapists themselves of being abusive, of creating the condition that causes him or her pain. At such a time, therapists must confront the abuse issue directly and support the patient's selective repression of memories that can overwhelm the patient if they emerge too quickly. Therapists must give permission for the patient to set boundaries between the unconscious and conscious processes, between the dream material and the waking thoughts, and between time in the past and time in the present.

A two-person team must provide protection at such a crucial stage of the patient's development and can do so by cessation of co-therapy treatment during the period of special vulnerability. It can be a stimulating factor in the patient's recognition of the abuse, but the problem remains of keeping the pace of the revelations of unconscious material to a manageable level. We find it fascinating that the rationale for Alfred Adler to employ multiple therapists in Vienna was the opportunity to break through a neurotic patient's resistance. Our co-therapy of higher functioning adults abused as children also follows the same rationale and allows them to break through their denial. However, in the case of Christine, the failure of her defenses led to a breakthrough of primary process material and consequent soaring anxiety. This was our first clue that Christine suffered from a borderline personality disorder. Modulating the unconscious revelations when her defenses suddenly collapsed became a major effort in treatment planning.

Christine continued to experience rising anxiety in group following her heightened awareness of sexual abuse in her past. The patient terminated the group in May 1986 stating, "I can't trust the group." Psychodynamically this constituted splitting between the bad mother, in the form of the group, and the abusive but trusted stepfather. The patient had split the group as she had split the therapists two months earlier.

### The Timing of Reparenting in Co-therapy Treatment

At the start of our co-therapy sessions in January 1986, we initiated reparenting work with Christine. Our reason for doing so was to give the patient new parenting messages and to help her restructure some of the ideas she had about herself. Some of the first messages were, "You are not alone," "You don't have to be perfect to be loved," and "It is OK for you to have needs." In retrospect, we believe the reparenting was begun prematurely. The patient's splitting prevented her from internalizing these messages. Christine was simply not able to respond to Vivian in a way that differentiated from her biological mother. The patient became increasingly intolerant of our clinical mistake and by March 1986 insisted that we shore up her defenses and terminate the co-therapy in the individual mode. The unconscious material was breaking through too rapidly for the patient to integrate it as part of her ego. The patient was correct in stopping the co-therapy yet continued to decompensate during the summer while in individual treatment with Bill.

During this period, the co-therapists changed their diagnosis from dependent personality disorder to borderline personality disorder. In August, Bill and the patient determined that she should be hospitalized. She remained in the hospital for three weeks. In October 1986, Christine returned to another of our co-led groups and continued individual treatment with Bill. It was the plan of the co-therapists to eschew co-therapy sessions in the individual mode in order to manage the emergence of primary process material stemming from the memories of abuse. Christine could tolerate co-therapy in the group because the group provided her with some distance from the co-therapy couple. The patient permitted herself to regress in the presence of Bill alone because in that context she had some assurance that the process could be controlled. Bill did not represent the hated stepfather at these times. The patient experienced a fusion with Bill's ego and borrowed generously from his identity in order to shore up her own. Analyzing the identity of a three-year-old child in one of her own dreams, Christine said, "I want the little girl whom I am nurturing to look like me. But for right now it's safer if she looks like you." Christine put her little girl into Bill for safekeeping, another expression of her projective identification. Christine also began her first primitive attempts at boundary formation, which consisted of dream images of containment and separateness. She remembered one dream of being on a beach where the waves had piled the sand high enough to separate her from the ocean and the whales who lived there. Christine identified Bill as one of the friendly whales and experienced a calmness in her dream. Bill had become the good mother.

In the presence of Vivian, Christine would not allow herself to be so vulnerable. She believed that the bad mother would attack her and projected that belief onto Vivian. Through 1987, we gradually included individual sessions with Vivian. Christine seemed less dependent on Bill. By October 1987, the patient was being treated five times a month by Bill and five times a month by Vivian. In November 1987, Christine requested a joint session with Bill and Vivian to talk to us before going on a date. She said, "I want to feel loved by both therapists." At the time we believed this was her acknowledgment of wanting two parents and wanting to initiate the reparenting contract. However, our expectations were still premature and were coloring our perception of what the patient was saying by her behavior. Vivian and Bill slowly began to realize that Christine was not ready to receive parenting of any kind from Vivian. During Bill's intensive individual treatment of her, he established a therapeutic alliance that allowed him to begin reparenting the patient. She was willing to listen and fight with him about her acting out and to test his competence and constancy as a person. Vivian had not established a therapeutic alliance with Christine, and therefore it was premature to attempt to reparent her. She would too easily dismiss or ignore Vivian as she would have her own mother. The therapeutic alliance allows the patient to go beyond transference and beyond projection to the establishment of a real relationship. Regressions are better understood by the patient and the therapist when the alliance is in place.

We have come to understand that a therapeutic alliance must be established with *both* therapists if successful treatment of the borderline patient is to be accomplished in co-therapy. It is most probable that the borderline patient cannot establish a therapeutic alliance with both therapists at once in the sense that other patients can. The therapist with whom the borderline patient first makes an alliance can initiate reparenting strategies with the patient, but the other co-therapist

cannot. Bill was impatient because Christine had not established a
therapeutic alliance with Vivian, and this degree of countertransference caused him to "encourage" Vivian and Christine to do so, much
to the dismay of Vivian and the anger of Christine. The patient had to
inform Bill with her anger before he could understand the inappropri-
ateness of his expectations.

As co-therapists we take considered steps to elucidate our countertransference and understand our participation in projective identification.

1. Therapists become aware.
2. Therapists take responsibility.
3. Therapists employ insight in the service of patient's treatment.
4. Therapists decide if and how much is appropriate to discuss with
   patient.

The following clinical material demonstrates these steps.

### Co-Therapist Help with Countertransference

In 1987, when Vivian was just beginning individual sessions with
Christine, Vivian forgot two appointments with her in less than one
month. Christine was angry. This occurrence was highly unusual
behavior on the part of Vivian, and Bill was immediately suspicious.
Together they discussed how and why Vivian forgot. They formulated
the following hypothesis: Christine projected disinterest onto Vivian
and chose Bill over Vivian as the parent with whom she could actively
engage herself. Vivian began her countertransference by feeling left
out. In Vivian's family of origin, Mother was chosen. "A child only
needs one parent, and that's Mother." Vivian responded to Christine's
aloofness by feeling not needed and acted-out unconsciously by
missing appointments. Christine's belief that she is not OK and that
women cannot be trusted was reinforced by Vivian's behavior. Thus,
both patient and therapist repeated family-of-origin issues.

Bill helped Vivian see why she would have forgotten the appointments. Because Vivian could trust Bill, she could look inside herself to
reveal her countertransference issue. Once Vivian understood her
countertransference, she became obliged to share the insight with the
patient. At their next appointment, Vivian said to Christine, "In my
family of origin, Mother is chosen. A child only needs one parent, and
that's Mother. You chose Bill over me as the involved parent, and I felt
left out. My forgetting was not your fault. I made a mistake."

Vivian must share the insight because it pertains directly to Christine and can help her correct a false impression of herself and other women. If the co-therapy team disagreed on this point, it might become a significant impediment to their ability to cooperate.

Christine's response appeared to prove the therapists' hypothesis correct. Following Vivian's talk with Christine, the client began to experience a new level of trust for her. Since the patient's mother would never admit mistakes, Vivian's candor proved helpful in differentiating Vivian from Mother. Mistakes are important with narcissistic patients also because of their tendency to idealize their therapists, as we shall demonstrate when we discuss Kevin.

### An Example of Projective Identification

In 1988, Christine called Vivian on the phone and said, "I'm angry at you and Bill. I'm back where I was two years ago!" Vivian listened and then asked, "Do you want to talk to Bill?" Christine came to the next co-therapy session angry at Vivian. Her anger resulted from her perception that Vivian did not want to deal with her when she had called on the phone the night before. She magnified her anger and turned it onto Bill when he raised the issue of competition, at which point both therapists and patient became confused. We suspected that unconscious dynamics were at work. Vivian suggested doing a psychodrama to reenact what had just happened.

BILL: Talk about the competition among the women of your family. Talk about grandmother who was most competitive of all.

CHRISTINE: No, I won't. Stop telling me what to do.

*(Vivian is silent.)*

Bill's interpretation is strangely incongruent with the context of the session, a suspicious sign of projective identification in Bion's view: ". . . there is a feeling that whatever else one has done, one has certainly not given a correct interpretation . . ." (Bion, 1959). In fact, talking with Vivian after the session, it became clear to Bill that he was projecting his own experience onto the patient.

Christine's stepfather no doubt interfered with arguments between her and her mother as a means to express his own hostility. Christine saw herself at fifteen years of age. She saw Bill as Stepfather abusing her, and she felt hateful and rageful. She saw Vivian as Mother remaining silent. This situation accurately recapitulated the patient's experience of her family of origin. Her stepfather was controlling and abusive. Her mother felt inadequate, depressed, and believed herself without power to protect either herself or her daughter. Christine appointed herself to protect the interests of both Mother and herself. Christine vented her rage and felt a subsequent loss of self-esteem.

In the psychodrama, each person was able to grasp the behavior that emerged unconsciously in the therapeutic session. Christine saw clearly her transference of Mother to Vivian and Stepfather to Bill. It was safer for her to express anger at Stepfather and to ignore Mother. A constant theme in Christine's nightmares had been the image of a woman with a knife cutting at Christine's throat. To direct rage at Mother was too frightening and too life threatening.

Following the session, the co-therapists consulted with each other to analyze their underlying participation and share their feelings. Bill saw clearly the projective identification occuring between Vivian and Christine. Christine projected her mother's powerlessness into Vivian, and she responded by appearing ineffective. Vivian saw clearly the projective identification occurring between Bill and Christine. Christine projected her stepfather's authoritarian ways into him, and Bill responded by becoming bossy.

The therapists were involved in an emotional drama that was not their own but the patient's. Once the dynamics of each participant in the co-therapy session was consciously understood by the therapists, they had a better grasp of what was going on when all three lapsed into unconscious behavior. When the roles emerge again in co-therapy, the therapists can call the process and refer to the psychodrama that all of them have enacted. The co-therapists "metabolized" (Langs, 1976) the harmful introject and Christine reinternalized it in a less threatening form and the patient learned the limits of her rage by this process. She will kill no one by it, and she herself will not be killed.


### More Countertransference


One borderline defense Christine employed was a dissociation from her body and her present surroundings. At these times, the patient lowered her head and averted her eyes downward. Sometimes she turned her head and body completely around so as to face the opposite direction. These occasions she referred to as "checking out." During an individual session with Vivian and Bill, in May 1988, Christine checked out and abruptly left the session. Later, she called Bill to set up an extra appointment. Vivian was not available, and he consented to meet with her alone. When Vivian learned of this, she remembered that something similar had occurred in group therapy earlier that month. Christine had "checked out" and had left the group room, and Bill had followed to continue therapy with her alone. During their absence a male member of the group had become angry and accused her of manipulation. He wanted Christine to remain with the members of the group and not take Bill away from them. When Christine returned, no one had confronted her—or Bill.

As a result of her insight, Vivian recognized that her silence in deference to the relationship between Christine and Bill was a manifestation of her countertransference. Vivian confronted Bill immediately. She pointed out that Bill was succumbing to manipulation and reinforcing the splitting by Christine. Bill had just ended his two-year treatment of Christine alone in individual therapy and he and Vivian had just begun a regular schedule of co-therapy treatment with Christine. Vivian interpreted Christine's manipulation as an unconscious attempt to restore the special bond she had experienced when she had individual sessions with him alone. Bill acknowledged his susceptibility to Christine's manipulation. He recognized that he did feel special in a relationship with a mentally ill woman because he had nurtured such a relationship with a woman in his own family of origin. Vivian and Bill agreed that the details of his countertransference should not be discussed with Christine because they were not pertinent to her treatment. They also agreed to take action in order to abate the patient's splitting. Bill met with Christine and empathically confronted her manipulation. Vivian joined them for the last fifteen minutes of the session. Christine responded to the confrontation with shame, which the co-therapists interpreted as her childhood feeling when she herself had been manipulated. She was prepared to return to the group with her new insight.

About this time, Christine had a dream that illustrated the psychodynamic impact of the co-therapy team. "In the dream, Bill was worried that Vivian had gone and wasn't coming back," she said. It became clear to Christine that her dream was a memory of the past. When she was two years old, her father had died and her mother had become severely depressed. In her dream, she projected her experience of abandonment onto Bill, and Vivian became the lost, beloved father. She included Vivian as a person loved by Bill. At an unconscious level she wished for a reunion with her dead father. Her identification with Bill let her see that she was capable of a loving relationship just as once upon a time she had loved her father and her father had loved her.

### Loss of the Special Bond

By June 1988, Christine complained that her sessions with Vivian stayed on the surface because she was afraid to regress. We agreed with Christine to proceed with co-therapy in all her individual sessions in

order to facilitate the depth of her work, although that meant the end of
individual sessions with Bill and a major emotional separation. As they
grieved the loss of the special bond that had been so important while
Christine borrowed parts of Bill's ego structure, the healing power of
projective identification was revealed. Over the next year, Bill shared
with Christine his feelings about her not needing him as intensely as
before. He entered a reverie for their lost closeness but differentiated
from the rage and fear of abandonment that Christine projected into
him. He spoke of separation as a process natural to all growth and
emphasized that he did not fear the loss of his self as a consequence. His
reverie assisted Christine to reintegrate her projections of rage and
abandonment in forms rationalized and depathologized by introspection.

### Why Co-Therapy Now?

Why was Christine able to accept co-therapy treatment in individual
therapy at this time? Emotionally speaking, the patient had grown up
to her teenage years and was now ready to receive the advantages of
dual transference. Her introject of the destructive mother was still
active but not as toxic as before. In co-therapy, which is now in
progress, Bill protects Christine's little girl self from the evil Mother
introject that she projects onto Vivian. For example, in one session,
when Christine's hatred and fear of Vivian emerged strongly, Bill
suggested that she externalize her emotions and visualize her mother.
She saw an evil witch on the chair. "I've always said there is something
I must get out of me, something that's making me sick," she said.
Christine recalled earlier memories of taking a knife and wanting to cut
herself and remove something from inside. She kept having associations with the past that she integrated with her present insight. She was
aware that cutting would not remove the hated introject. She is now
more aware of her projections and gains successive insights without
borderline regressions.

At last, we discovered a reparenting role for Vivian. Christine
needed Vivian to mother her teenage self. In this role, Vivian listens to
her talk about being with men and her excitement and wildness.
Christine began one session saying, "I'm having trouble being sexual."
She related a dream. "I was hiding from a man and woman, and I was
hiding at the woman's house. I'm confused. I have no idea of my sex or
who I am supposed to be." The patient became aware that her identity
as a woman was not fully developed. She began a contract with Vivian
to assist her in feeling powerful and confident in that respect.

The patient now understands the specific kind of reparenting she needs from each therapist, and the therapists are now able to respond appropriately. This was nearly three years after our premature attempt to reparent a borderline patient in co-therapy.

## KEVIN

Kevin, a highly narcissistic personality, was initially interviewed and treated by Vivian. The patient had a false start in his course of individual treatment with Vivian, attending twenty sessions in 1980 and then not returning to treatment until 1983. In December of that year, he entered group therapy with Vivian and a male co-therapist. Group therapy was indicated to help the patient overcome his isolation. The presence of a male co-therapist permitted the patient a modicum of safety, since he projected so much negative mother energy onto Vivian. The male co-therapist was able to confront with humor the patient's long, attention-seeking soliloquies and accompanying hyperbole. The co-therapy treatment succeeded in letting the patient experience a bond with the male therapist. In March 1984, Kevin lost his first male co-therapist who was replaced by Bill. He had no other therapy besides his weekly group. From March 1984 to August 1986, the co-therapy treatment of Kevin was not effective. The patient established a therapeutic alliance with Vivian but not with Bill. He obsessed about his conflictual relationship with his mother and repeated stories of his childhood endlessly to the group. He did not progress.

Kevin projected his mother onto the group-as-a-whole and saw them disapproving his behavior. Efforts of the co-therapists to interpret this phenomenon fell on deaf ears. He was not able to listen to group members and failed to empathize with their struggles. This condition exacerbated to the point where he terminated the group prematurely in August 1986. He was so incensed that he did not follow the protocol for people terminating group. Rather, he avoided termination issues and did not allow the group to process his leaving. In this manner he fulfilled the function of a classic scapegoat by making himself a target for the others in the group and eventually choosing to exclude himself completely. As the Scapegoat Leader (see Emerging Leaders, Appendix), he perpetuated a pattern of social isolation that he had been repeating for many years.

### How Co-Therapists Collaborate to Manage Their Countertransference

When Kevin left treatment, he angrily denounced the group for the many ways it had mistreated him with unsupportive criticism.

KEVIN: I'm fed up with how I'm treated here. No one understands me. No one believes I can be happy by choosing a wife. I'm leaving.

GROUP: Come on, Kevin. How realistic is an Asian mail bride? You couldn't make it to Italy for a vacation without overwhelming anxiety; how are you going to make it to Thailand?

KEVIN: You're not supporting me. I'm very anxious now. You're not giving me the help I need. You don't give me the kind of attention I want. I don't think this group has helped me at all. I might as well go.

Following the group, the co-therapists discussed their countertransference reactions to the patient's leaving and his vehement devaluation of the group. Bill's defensive reaction was one of happiness and relief. There were many narcissistic males in his family-of-origin, and one less was good riddance. Vivian's countertransference was expressed by her sadness. She recalled her father leaving each evening and her childhood belief that she must not be good enough for him to stay. By their candid and open discussion, the co-therapists were able to put in perspective their unique countertransference reactions and come to a new understanding that separated the patient's issues from their own personal dynamics. In this example, the co-therapy team provided an emotional buffer for the considerable amount of anger the narcissistic patient puts on therapists. This has proven to be true with the borderline patient as well.

The co-therapy team was careful to discuss with Kevin's group the distortions of the patient's projections so that they could cope with their own sense of being devalued. We did err as a co-therapy team because we failed to function at maximum capacity. One of us could have supported Kevin and his grandiosity while the other remained skeptical. In that way, we could have avoided collusion with other group members in driving out the scapegoat.

Countertransference with the narcissistic patient can be intense. We were often annoyed by Kevin's devaluation of the therapy process. He would attribute his criticisms of therapy to "friends" rather than directly facing us with his anger. He would call on the phone and announce in exaggerated tones how badly he was doing. Since Bill had a number of narcissistic persons in his own family of origin, Vivian was helpful in pointing out how that vitiated his patience with Kevin. Bill's countertransference emerged as a difficulty listening to the patient's verbal output. In his own family of origin, his defensive strategy with narcissistic family members had been to assume a posture of listening without really doing so. Since that would repeat what the patient experienced in his own family and fulfill his expectation to be rejected, Bill's renewed attention to listening proved to be an essential component of effective treatment. Vivian's gentle reminders assisted Bill to be a better listener.

Following Kevin's departure from group, the co-therapists treated the patient once in December 1986. It was clear that he was decompensating and experiencing the acute loneliness that he had so long concealed from himself by his defensive actions. The patient was hospitalized with a major affective disorder in January 1987 for three weeks. He returned to co-therapy in group treatment in February of that year. As part of his post-hospital treatment plan, he began a course of individual psychotherapy with Bill, twice a month.

In retrospect, we believe that Kevin should have been in a course of individual treatment during his two years of group therapy prior to hospitalization. However, we did not challenge the client's resistance when he protested that he could not afford more psychotherapy. This was an expression of countertransference that neither co-therapist realized at the time. Both therapists were influenced by his devaluation of therapy and did not encourage him to do more. Vivian's reluctance to recommend individual treatment strongly was stimulated by Kevin's miserly attitudes. In her family, it was considered admirable to spend very little money on oneself. Bill's resistance stemmed from a wish to starve his own narcissistic self. From that point of view, Kevin did not deserve the nurturing gift of therapy. The hospital staff recommended both individual and group therapy for Kevin following his discharge and thereby called into consciousness the countertransference of the co-therapists. Our example illustrates a basic truth: countertransference to which both co-therapists are blind must be pointed out by an outside source. We suspect that unrecognized and unanalyzed countertransference accounts for why many patients leave treatment.

### How Co-Therapy Facilitated Kevin's Changes in Group

The co-therapy team treated Kevin only in group therapy, and we perceive his greatest improvement by the way he has changed in relation to his group. The following incidents demonstrate how the co-therapy team facilitated Kevin's changes.

In February 1987, a therapeutic turning point occurred when Bill insisted that Kevin look at the relationship with his father. Vivian was clear that this was not the salient point but trusted Bill's intuition. The maneuver was felicitous because it did divert the patient's attention from his obsession with his mother. This is one example of the diversity that our team brings to the treatment of a narcissistic personality. Many times the patient cannot please both transference objects because they hold contradictory views. In this way, the co-therapy team is able to create a positive double bind for the patient. The patient must therefore find a way to please himself. This is a novel problem for the narcissist, whose injunction "Don't be you" (Goulding & Goulding, 1978) comes from his narcissistic mother. Each therapist in the co-therapy team must establish a therapeutic alliance with the patient, and each therapist will accomplish that differently. The maneuver did allow Bill to make a therapeutic alliance with Kevin because the patient saw that he could make a healthy relationship with Bill, whereas he could not with his own father.

During the course of individual therapy with Bill, Kevin experienced the insight that his father was not ideal. A mistake Bill committed during one session facilitated his insight. Bill had forgotten how to operate the tape recorder, and Kevin discovered he knew more about this than the therapist. Armed with the knowledge that Bill could make mistakes, Kevin diminished the degree of splitting between his mother and father and the frequency with which he resorted to that primitive defense.

It is significant to note that Vivian had been recommending that Kevin desist speaking of his mother since 1985. Kevin needed to hear from the male therapist, "Talk about your father." Whereas Kevin could not hear Vivian above the voice of his mother in his head, Bill's message about Father came through on a clear channel. Once Kevin ceased obsessing about his mother, he was able to have a better picture of himself, his feelings, and what he wanted. Figuratively, he is turning down the volume of his mother's voice and is better able to listen to others in his group. His capacity for empathy in the group grows as his capacity to care and empathize with himself increases.

Bill began individual treatment of Kevin in February 1987. The course of treatment included body therapy, a procedure in which the patient focused on his awareness of his own body by means of a series of breathing and relaxation exercises. In contrast with Christine, Kevin was able to use body work effectively as a means to greater integration of the self. The therapists do not initiate body work with a borderline patient because the boundaries between self and others are so tenuous. The body work produced twofold results. First, the patient was able to stop his obsessing and second, the patient was able to give himself a generous amount of self-stroking. As Kevin's ability to accept strokes improved, so Bill's nurturing was felt more deeply and internalized by the patient. This permitted the patient to perceive Bill as a nurturing father and begin to rely on him when he needed emotional supplies.

About this time Kevin had a dream that illustrated his growing acceptability to the group in contrast to his family of origin. "My father was in a big house that was messed up. I wanted things to be different, so I went to another house and was surprised to find how easy it was to get in. I went to the kitchen where everyone had gathered around the table as if I was going to say something." Kevin also decreased the extent to which he exaggerated his statements to the group. He no longer believed it was necessary in order to obtain the group's attention. His pouting and other behavior that mimicked his mother diminished as he relinquished her attention-seeking maneuvers. The group recognized his new-found directness and genuineness and responded by liking him more. They were gratified by his questions and comments that showed his interest in them. He shifted from the Parent ego state to the Adult ego state in asking members questions about themselves and shifted into the Child ego state in sharing about himself. When in the Parent ego state, he is more often in Nurturing Parent than Critical Parent (Berne, 1961). As his dream implied he had created a new family for himself.

### Reparenting

The co-therapy strategy of reparenting developed slowly. Reparenting began when the co-therapists encouraged Kevin to work with Bill. This was a difficult decision for Kevin to make because in his family of origin, he had to relinquish his desire to be close to Father and fuse with Mother. Had Vivian competed with Bill as the therapist of choice, the co-therapy team would have repeated the drama of the original triad: Mother intrudes, Father avoids, and Kevin languishes. In reparenting, co-therapy teams must be careful not to replicate the pathology of the family of origin.

Kevin's ability to utilize reparenting messages is illustrated by the following. When the patient experienced an anxiety attack in which his punitive superego made mincemeat of his ego, he would say to himself the internalized message, "Bill wouldn't want me to feel this way." His statement reflects an intermediate stage in the reparenting process. The messages are still attributed to the therapist and have not become completely integrated with the patient's ego. It is important to remember that the narcissistic personality will hear this message as a criticism unless he has a therapeutic alliance with his therapist and feels that the therapist empathically understands his pain. For this reason Bill devoted much time to empathic interpretations of Kevin's behavior. Interpretations of this kind would be pointless with Christine because they would not serve to confront the destructiveness of her acting out. The act of confrontation allows the borderline patient to arrive at the awareness herself, whereas interpretation by the therapist would only invite resistance.

A turning point for Kevin occurred in group when he became aware of his jealousy with respect to Christine's relationship to Bill in group. Vivian asked the question, "What are you jealous about, Kevin?" Kevin became aware that he too wanted the nurturing from Bill that Christine was receiving. Vivian's gambit was well placed, because Kevin needed permission from Mother to be close to Father. This was at variance with the system in Kevin's family of origin: Brother gets love from Father, and Kevin must seek love from his unloving mother. Kevin reacted with bewilderment because Vivian's question exposed his desire for closeness and his belief that he was not capable of it. With the encouragement of Vivian and the group, he chose to explore closeness with Bill, including sitting next to him.

All members of our groups have the option to request that Vivian or Bill hold them. The reparenting contracts we have with Christine and Kevin also include our holding them at their request. Bill developed an exceptional agreement with Kevin so that Bill can demonstrate his affection spontaneously as he feels close to Kevin. They agreed to this arrangement to reinforce Kevin's perception of himself and his life as real and genuine, including the affection and strokes he receives. Demonstrating spontaneous affection would not work with Christine because of her need to maintain a clear boundary with both therapists.

Interestingly, Vivian's reparenting contract with Kevin specifies that she cannot be too involved with him. His mother was so intrusive that Kevin wants Vivian to maintain her boundaries with respect to him, both physically and emotionally. That means he approaches her when he wants contact. Kevin's self-image was fused with that of his mother, and therefore, he needs distance in his relationship with Vivian in order to heal the narcissistic wounds. Bill strokes Kevin, while Vivian keeps a respectful distance from him. A solo therapist cannot accomplish both tasks simultaneously.

It is also significant to note that the reparenting was first begun with the male co-therapist because the patient was simply too much involved with his own biological mother. An attempt by Vivian to initiate reparenting messages would simply have been mistaken and would have met with stiff competition from the mother introject embedded in Kevin's ego. Now that the patient has established a loving bond with Bill, he is better able to return both to the issue of mothering and to his need for an adequate mother who reflects and mirrors his aspirations realistically and does not intrude on his identity.

The reparenting strategy of a distant and friendly mother has borne fruit. Kevin used to complain angrily to Vivian as he had to his own mother in a futile attempt to gain his mother's attention. Like a mirror, he had reflected his mother's anger and neglected his own feelings. Now he can look at Vivian and experience his own feelings of sadness because Vivian does not contaminate Kevin with her own feelings. Kevin's relationship with Bill, as the loving father, is secure. He can return to Vivian with full knowledge that Bill will accept his desire to be close to Mother.

### Concluding Remarks on Co-Therapy Treatment with Christine and Kevin

During splitting, the therapists were careful not to support the patient's negative perception of the co-therapist. A good relationship between the co-therapists is necessary to do this. Feelings of competition will undermine this.

Due to Christine's splitting between Vivian and Bill, we had to build on the trust that she had for Bill before proceeding with co-therapy. As a way to accomplish this, she entered treatment with him alone in individual therapy after she left group. To continue co-therapy with the patient in the individual mode would serve only to increase the likelihood of the patient splitting between the co-therapists.

The roles we take in the treatment of the patients depend a great deal on the dynamics of each patient. For example, in both clients described above, Bill established the reparenting contract first. This does not indicate Vivian's aversion to do so; rather, it reflects the relative ease with which both persons entered into relationships with males. Christine felt a hatred and distrust of women, and Kevin devalued them.

We chose co-therapy treatment of Christine in the individual mode because in our clinical judgment Christine needed to form a bond with both male and female parental figures. Christine formed the bonds after she worked through her negative transference of abusive Stepfather and neglectful Mother. As Mintz asserts and we quote above, Christine needed the protection of one therapist as she worked through her vehement transference with the other. In contrast, we did not offer co-therapy treatment to Kevin in the individual mode because he needed the distance from the female parental figure. Co-therapy treatment in the group provided him that distance (Roller & Shaskan, 1982).

# PART II

# Master Practitioners

# • 7 •

# *Phases of Co-Therapy Team Development*

## JAMES M. DUGO and ARIADNE P. BECK

### INTRODUCTION

Like all living systems, co-therapy relationships evolve. This chapter describes the phases in the development of that evolution. As supervisors of co-leaders and as co-leaders ourselves for ten years, we have been powerfully struck by the profound implications of that evolution for co-leadership potential at any particular phase, for client development and for the dynamics of the group-as-a-whole. Though not alone in noticing this fact, we offer in this chapter a more comprehensive and detailed look at these implications (Benjamin, 1972; McMahon & Links, 1984).

We come from a base in systems theory, developmental theory, and from a set of values informed by a humanistic focus on personal and relationship emergence. We have formulated a model of the phases of development of the co-therapy relationship that addresses tasks, goals, and structural, stylistic, and qualitative dimensions of the co-therapy relationship. In addition, it spells out the implications of the co-therapy process for individual clients and for the group-as-a-whole. Further, it traces the mutual impact of the co-leadership team and the institution,

James M. Dugo, Ph.D., is a clinical psychologist in private practice in Chicago and a member of the core faculty of the Forest Institute of Professional Psychology, Wheeling, Illinois.

Ariadne P. Beck, M.A., is a psychologist in private practice in Indian Head Park and Des Plaines, Illinois. She is coordinator of the Chicago Group Development Research Team.

solo, or group private practice within which the team functions. The model highlights the isomorphy of processes that is a characteristic of all complex living systems. (In systems theory the idea of isomorphy postulates that beneath the diversity of content between systems there are identical structures and organizing processes [Cooper, 1976; Durkin, 1981]). Admittedly, fully spelling out this model is an ambitious endeavor covering a broad spectrum of issues, none of which can be developed in depth in this chapter. Our experience with co-therapy is in the group therapy context. Our assumption is that these phases and issues apply to co-leaders who work with families, couples, or individuals as well.

The central focus here is on phase-specific issues as the evolution of the informal aspects of a co-leader pair is tracked through the first three of nine possible phases of development. The focus on the first three phases was chosen because many co-therapy relationships are formed for relatively brief periods of time and do not, therefore, have the opportunity to evolve into the later phases. Second, we believe that co-therapists who can evolve to at least the third phase begin to prove the maxim that the sum is greater than its parts. Third, we have observed that groups do not achieve a higher phase of development than the one that the co-therapists have achieved, and therefore, it is desirable to move past the stress and competitiveness of Phase 2 as efficiently as possible. In this chapter we describe a positive approach to the issues of each phase and indicate briefly the consequences of failures to cope with issues at each point. There is an assumption inherent in our work: that the best co-therapy is done by partners who make a commitment to an ongoing relationship, who reason with each other, and who accept responsibility to work on the evolution of that relationship.

Given the level of "noise" that occurs in the life of a group, it is important to have a model for thinking about and making sense out of what is happening. This is important not only to make a leader feel better but also to allow him or her to intervene with a combined use of intuition and reason. We have been working with and further elaborating Beck's nine-phase theory of group development, which describes the evolution of group structure and emerging leadership, as a way of making sense out of the noise in the group-as-a-whole (Beck, 1974, 1981a, 1981b; Beck, Dugo, Eng, & Lewis, 1986). Four leadership roles emerge early in a group's life and evolve over the course of the nine phases of group development (Beck & Peters, 1981; Beck, Eng, & Brusa, 1989; Peters & Beck, 1982). By analyzing groups from this perspective, our attention has been drawn to the parallels between impasses in group process (which can occur at any stage of group develpment) and impasses in the co-therapy team. For those who are not familiar with this theory, a brief description of the nine phases of group development and the four emergent leadership roles appear in the Appendix of this book.

In the last 15 years a number of articles have proposed developmental frameworks specifically for understanding and organizing how co-leadership relationships evolve (Brent & Marine 1982; Dicks et al., 1980; Gallogly & Levine 1979; McMahon & Links, 1984; Winter, 1976). All of the articles outline from four to six phases in the evolution of the co-therapy relationship. Also, all of the articles suggest that the quality of evolution of the co-therapists' relationship has important implications for the effectiveness of the treatment process. Two of the papers validate the necessity that co-therapy teams should evolve past the early phases for them to be more effective than a single therapist (Dick et al., 1980; Gallogly & Levine, 1979). It seems that as co-therapists are developing in the early phases of becoming a team, they are often pulling in different directions or hesitating to assert their leadership. Piper et al. (1979), although not directly addressing phase development, found that the degree to which co-therapists were consistent in their focus was related to higher percentages of quality patient work and positive outcome at statistically significant levels.

Group members may get contradictory messages in the early phases of co-therapy team development and splitting and subgrouping are common results. It is only when a co-therapy team has evolved through the early phases that the sum of their efforts is greater than what one leader can do alone. This raises a number of important concerns. At the most basic level: Are co-leaders useful in all settings? Are there methods to shorten the time of working through the early phases? What are the implications for the group-as-a-whole, the patients, or the institution when the co-therapy team is at different phases of development?

The general purpose of this model is to help co-leaders become more aware of the dimensions in the development of a co-therapy relationship so that, first, the process can be more explicit; second, there is a model to help guide co-leaders and agencies in setting up and conducting co-treatment arrangements; third, that co-leaders can begin to see more clearly the parallel and interactive aspects among the development of the co-therapy relationship, the development of the group-as-a-whole, and the development of the individuals in the group. Table 1 describes briefly the nine phases of co-therapy team development.

The developmental phases track the structural evolution of the relationship. As indicated earlier, there is a parallel structural evolution in the group-as-a-whole (Dugo & Beck, 1985). At some time in the future our intent is to trace the impact of the co-therapy phases of development on the phases of development of the group-as-a-whole.

To place our nine-phase theory into the context of the existing literature cited above, we have prepared Table 2 showing the parallels

## TABLE 1. Nine Phases of Co-therapy Team Development

*Phase 1: Creating a contract*

In this phase the co-leaders establish a foundation by creating some formal norms for the critical aspects of their relationship and for the conduct of the group. Also, the way in which they each conceptualize and process the individual and group dynamics is addressed. Possible role differentiations may begin to be explored. The degree of explicitness or implicitness of the contract determines the degree of ease or clarity with which the co-therapy team proceeds.

*Phase 2: Forming an identity*

The basic task for co-therapists is to establish an initial identity as a team and to form the structure of their relationship. This generates competitive feelings, irritations, differences in personal and conceptual priorities, and the temptation to resolve conflict by the use of power or manipulation. These competitive issues must be resolved and norms generated that will allow collaborative effort to begin. The co-therapists are challenged to identify issues, clarify feelings, and negotiate a structure that is respectful of both diverging and converging elements in their viewpoints and personalities.

*Phase 3: Building a team*

Having settled basic structural issues in order to begin a true working relationship, the co-therapists begin to learn about the range and depth of each others' intuitions, conceptual orientation, and intervention skills as these apply to the clinical realities of individual and group dynamics. Learning about each other is becoming a reality while learning from each other is becoming a possibility. Mutual respect is established in this process. A jointly determined style of co-leadership and communication in the group is worked out during this phase.

*Phase 4: Developing closeness*

The co-therapists are establishing a deeper interest and attraction based on an actual working knowledge of one another. This process leads to emerging feelings of closeness and attraction, on sexual and other levels. The ways in which closeness is acknowledged and boundaries are established become central features of this phase. The potential of the relationship as a context for growth and change becomes apparent.

*Phase 5: Defining strengths and limitations*

The important task of this phase is for the co-therapists to develop realistic perceptions of their strengths and limitations in their own relationship and as therapists in the group. This process stimulates the emergence of underlying needs and leads to intense feelings that if not discussed and clarified, can trigger acting-out behavior. A new commitment to a deeper understanding of themselves and each other emerges from this struggle.

*Phase 6: Exploring possibilities*

There is a reworking of the co-therapy contract that allows for exploratory new behavior as persons and greater flexibility in role behavior as therapists in the group. This stage is often a conflict-free period of personal exploration and readjustment of the working relationship.

*(cont.)*

**TABLE 1** *(cont.)*

*Phase 7: Supporting self-confrontation*
Therapists take responsibility to challenge their own personal and professional frontiers confronting the issues that interfere with growth. Regressive aspects of these explorations can either be addressed or acted-out, depending on the leaders' awareness and ability to confront self-defeating behavior. The mutual support of this process, even when it is difficult, characterizes this phase.

*Phase 8: Integrating and implementing changes*
The personal insights and changes resulting from the self-confrontations in Phase 7 must now be integrated. Most likely this will lead to changes both personally and professionally and may necessitate a redefinition of the team as well as other dimensions of their relationship. A major task of Phase 8 then involves decisions about continuing to work together and/or supporting each other in the development of new ventures.

*Phase 9: Closing*
The need for closure exists whether the change at this point is a termination or a redefinition of the co-therapy relationship or of its tasks. A healthy transition requires an acknowledgement to the partner of his or her significance in the shared process prior to the change and a review of what was and was not accomplished.

and differences. We have placed each phase from each existing theory of co-therapy development in the row that corresponds to the comparable phase in our own scheme. There is a column for each theorist, and the numbers in parentheses are those given by that author to that phase.

In reviewing Table 2 we see a general agreement on the first two phases and on some form of termination phase. All but one theory identified our Phase 3; one theory identified our Phase 4, and one our Phase 5. One theory added a grieving phase that we did not explicitly discuss. We believe these theories are based on the fact that most co-therapy relationships are not long term and do not have the opportunity to evolve to later phases. The on-going co-therapy relationship does exist, however, primarily in private practice and in hospital settings that have stable psychiatric outpatient or inpatient teams. The fact that there is a high agreement on the first three phases may also reflect both the necessity for co-therapy teams to evolve to this cooperative work phase in order to be effective and the difficulties commonly experienced in achieving this goal.

In the rest of this chapter we focus exclusively on the first three phases in the evolution of a co-therapy relationship between therapists of relatively equal levels of experience and knowledge with groups, that is, therapists who are perceived by their groups as sharing the task leadership role fairly equally. We believe our theory also applies to

**TABLE 2. Theories of Co-Therapy Development**[a]

| Dugo and Beck (1985) | McMahon & Links (1984) | Brent & Marine (1982) | Dick et al. (1980) | Gullogly & Levine (1979) | Winters (1976) |
|---|---|---|---|---|---|
| Creating a contract (1) | Endorsing the co-therapy pair (1) | Encounter (1) | Formation (1) | Parallel phase (1) | Encounter (1) |
| Forming an identity (2) | Testing phase (2) | Power and control (2) | Development (2) | Authority (2) | Differentiation conflict norm (2) |
| Building a cooperative team (3) | Role clarification (3) | | Stabilization (3) | Intimacy (3) | Production (3) |
| Developing closeness (4) | | Intimacy (3) | | | |
| Defining strengths and limitations (5) | Individuation (4) | | | | |
| Exploring possibilities (6) | | | | | |
| Supporting self-confrontation (7) | | | | | |
| Integrating & implementing changes (8) | | | | | |
| Closing reorganization (9) | Termination (5) | Separation (4) | Refreshment (4) | Separation/termination (4) | Separation (4) |
| | | | | | Grieving rejoining (6) |

[a]Each phase from each existing theory of co-therapy development has been placed in the same row as the Dugo and Beck phase with which the content coincides substantively.

nequipos and co-learners as defined in Chapter 2 of this book. However, the implications for clients, group, and organization are somewhat different at each phase. This chapter simply does not allow us to elaborate that development. We shall describe the critical issues to be addressed at each phase of the emergent co-therapy relationship. Then we shall explore the corresponding implications of these issues for the co-therapy relationship itself, for individual clients, for the group-as-a-whole, and for the institution or group private practice within which they work (McMahon & Links, 1984). When we refer to critical issues, we mean the relationship-level tasks at each phase of the process. These are the issues that naturally arise at a given developmental point and that the co-therapists must address and work out if their partnership is to continue to grow and develop.

Any relationship has both formal and informal aspects. Our theory describes the evolution of the informal relationship between co-leaders and the interface between the informal and formal aspects. The formal aspects begin with the profession, level of experience, and the role that each co-leader fills in the organization or group private practice in which they will conduct their group. The policies of the organization will also determine the location and time of the group, the way clients are selected and how fees are charged, the supervision requirements, the coordination with individual or other therapies, whether testing is done, whether the group is audio or video recorded and whether or not there are observers of the group. To the extent that these formal dimensions are not determined by the context, as in individual private practice, they become important issues to be addressed by the co-leaders before the group begins.

The informal aspects of the co-therapy relationship have been organized into seven major issues. The nine-phase theory and the identification of seven issues initially emerged empirically from an examination of our own co-therapy relationship. As each phase was discussed, we then drew on our extensive experiences in supervising other co-leaders and in co-leading with other colleagues. As we worked, the two major dimensions of the dyadic relationship itself and the relationship of the dyad to the group emerged. The seven issues emerged naturally as we attempted to specify the important aspects of the process of becoming a team. The seven issues are not entirely separate from each other; in fact, they build on each other. We felt, however, that each of them is significant enough to require an investment of time and effort from the co-therapists. Each of these issues also has the potential (at different times in the developmental sequence) of becoming a stumbling block to the overall evolution of the relationship.

A review of the literature subsequent to our own analysis confirmed the prominence of those seven issues. Therefore, we have indicated relevant references after each of the seven issues. The literature suggests that ease of communication and compatibility of orientation and style of leadership have been focused on the most, possibly reflecting that these are key factors in the co-therapy relationship.

In the list of seven issues we have italicized one word that will be used throughout the chapter to remind the reader of the substantive focus of each issue. In each of the nine phases, the following seven issues need to be addressed if the co-therapy relationship is fully to develop its potential. The first four are dyadic relationship issues:

1. The *attraction* and appeal experienced by the co-leaders in relation to each other (Rabin, 1967).
2. The *gains* to be achieved personally and professionally from the relationship and from doing the group together (Heilfron, 1969).
3. The ease of *communication* and degree of defensiveness in the relationship (Block, 1961; Davis & Lohr, 1971; Dies, Mallett, & Johnson, 1979; Williams, 1976).
4. The *negotiation* of the partnership contract and the commitment to regularly examine the relationship and the quality of the collaboration (Lothstein, 1979; Sager & Kaplan, 1972; Williams, 1976).

The remaining three are co-therapist–group issues:

5. The degree of *compatibility* of orientations as therapists and of style of leadership (Gans, 1962; Lundin & Arnov, 1952; Paulson, Burroughs, & Gelb, 1977; Solomon, Loeffler, & Frank, 1953; Williams, 1976).
6. The evolution of client-to-therapist(s) *bonding* and the co-leaders' views of this process (Getty & Shannon, 1969).
7. The *stresses* that result from the evolution of the co-therapy relationship in juxtaposition to the evolution of the particular group being led; differences in the roles where co-therapists work; and events in their personal lives (Lothstein, 1980; McGee & Schuman, 1970).

All of these issues address important and changing dimensions of the way co-therapists function together. The first four address aspects of their own dyadic relationship, and the last three address the ways in which they conceptualize and proceed as a therapeutic team in relation to individual clients and the group-as-a-whole. Each of these seven issues has a unique significance within each of the nine phases. In addition these issues carry implications for the individual clients, the group-as-a-whole, and the organization within which the therapists work.

As co-therapists participate in group, they vary in their level of activity and intervention. The task leadership role can be shared by co-therapists who are perceived by their group as relatively equal in skill and experience and who are sufficiently active to share the responsibility. When therapists are of unequal experience or skill, it is rare that they are both perceived by their group as Task Leaders in guiding the structural development of the group. There are also groups in which the designated leader is too inactive in the process of the group to fulfill the task leadership role. In these instances (i.e., Tavistock groups; certain psychoanalytic groups, etc.) a member emerges who fulfills the within-group aspects of the role. We describe below the seven issues and their implications for each of the relationships as they are expressed in the first three phases of development of a co-therapy relationship.

## PHASE 1: CREATING A CONTRACT

Preferably this phase begins before the leaders formally start their group. They begin to work out the basic norms for how the critical issues of creating a co-leadership relationship will be negotiated. In this phase the co-leaders establish a foundation by creating some formal norms for the critical aspects of their relationship and for the conduct of the group. Also, the way in which each conceptualizes and processes individual and group dynamics will be addressed. Possible role differentiations may begin to be explored. The degree of explicitness or implicitness of the contract determines the degree of ease or clarity with which the co-therapy team proceeds. This phase sets a model for the quality and thoroughness of future interactions.

### The Seven Issues as Expressed in Phase 1

*PHASE 1 Dyadic Relationship Issues*

*Issue 1. Attraction:* The degree of attraction and appeal experienced by the co-leaders toward each other strongly determines how meaningful their relationship can be. It is the basis for the initial bonding between partners and influences how much motivation they each have for pursuing the relationship. In addition, it is the initial base for both the quality and kind of trust that develop between them. The attraction and appeal may be experienced on any one of a number of different personal or professional levels.

*Issue 2. Gains:* Each partner clarifies what he or she wants and hopes to get from the relationship, both personally and professionally, in the context of co-leading a group. It is important for co-therapists to share these goals and expectations with each other because they contribute to the meaning of the relationship and determine the type of bond that the two people will form. In sharing these goals and expectations, the opportunity is created for some amount of negotiation to take place. This begins to ground the relationship, allowing a realistic appraisal of what can be accomplished given the constraints at the time. Reaching agreement on this level of the partnership heightens the degree of motivation of the partners to continue to work on the relationship openly and influences the quality of trust that develops between them over time.

*Issue 3. Communication:* The ease of communication and the degree of competitiveness in the co-therapy relationship have been reflected in the previous two issues but deserve attention in their own right. This dimension affects all aspects of the relationship and of the group as well. Major consequences of the quality of communication in the contracting phase are that it tends to determine how accurately the co-leaders present themselves and therefore how accurately they are able to get to know one another.

*Issue 4. Negotiation:* The explicit negotiation of the partnership contract generates an atmosphere that makes the clarification of rules about the group and about the relationship desirable. A commitment is needed to examine the relationship and the quality of the collaboration regularly. The most common errors that co-leaders make in approaching their joint work is failing to realize the amount of time it takes to do the job effectively. Even when time is quite limited, as in inpatient settings, a quick 15-minute check through the first four issues will enhance the quality of the leadership experience. A frequent review of all seven issues will help co-leaders negotiate their concerns while the group is in process. In addition, the more a leader reviews these issues in his or her own mind and articulates them to others, the quicker and more effective the negotiation process will become.

*PHASE 1 Co-Therapist–Group Issues*

*Issue 5. Compatibility:* It is important for co-leaders to explore the compatibility of their therapeutic orientations and styles of leadership. Whether or not it is clearly formulated, every therapist has a theoretical base from which he or she operates. Every therapist also has a characteristic style of relating and intervening and usually believes that these two things are integrated or at least coordinated with each other. However, personality and degree of self-awareness strongly interact with situational factors and sometimes lead to behavior that does not fit with either the theory or the expectations the therapist has expressed. Because this is true of everyone, it is especially important in the co-therapy relationship for the partners to be willing to share their orientations with each other and explore any areas of difference that might lead them to work at odds with each other or where they might have difficulty in supporting each others' efforts. It is also important to establish the kind of communication that will allow each of them to give feedback to the other regarding discrepancies between goals and actions in the group itself.

*Issue 6. Bonding:* The two therapists must address their views of the evolution of client-to-therapist bonding. This is complicated by any relationship that either therapist has with any particular client outside of the group. However, co-therapy to some degree means sharing responsibility for clients and sharing involvement with clients. How that is defined and carried out strongly determines the degree of competitiveness that evolves between co-leaders and the way they begin to think about and process issues of competition about clients.

*Issue 7. Stresses:* Co-therapists have an ongoing responsibility to make known to each other the stresses that are affecting their lives and their relationship. These stresses may emanate from experiences in the group, in the organization or private practice in which they work, or in their personal lives. Time must be allotted to share and process events, and rules must be set for negotiating the explicit and implicit ways in which these events impact their interactions and their feelings about each other.

Each of these issues has ramifications in the experiences of individual clients and in the process of the group-as-a-whole. In the next section, we describe the implications of these issues in the same sequence in which the issues have been presented above.

## PHASE 1 Dyadic Relationship Issues: Implications for Clients and Group-as-a-Whole

*Issue 1. Attraction:* The members of a group observe the co-therapists' relationship in great detail and are sensitive to both obvious and subtle aspects of their interaction or lack of interaction. The bond that the co-leaders develop between them becomes a model to each client for his or her involvement with other group members, the therapists, and potentially for relationships outside the group.

The felt sense of interest and attraction of the co-therapy team and their ability to transfer that interest to the group as a joint endeavor set the tone for the investment of clients in the group and influence their willingness to allow the group to have an impact on them. It is important, therefore, that co-leaders let a group know that they have a strong sense of involvement in each other and in the group process if they expect similar commitments from group members.

*Issue 2. Gains:* Therapists' willingness to clarify openly personal and professional expectations leads to a high level of trust between them. This is also the major single influence on the trust level that clients try to achieve among themselves and with the therapists. Participation in a group for purposes of change arouses anxiety regarding trust in any member. For clients who are in crisis or suffering from severe emotional disturbances, this can be an overwhelming issue. It would be difficult to exaggerate the significance of this one dimension of the co-therapy relationship and its impact on the therapeutic alliance with clients.

Energy that co-therapists invest in their own relationship is generative for them: that is, it does not drain them—it tends to rejuvenate them. One major consequence of that availability of energy in the team is that group-level issues are more likely to be recognized and addressed. It is our view that group-level issues are the most difficult for leaders to see in the moment they occur and to manage in a collaborative manner.

*Issue 3. Communication:* The degree of openness between co-leaders directly affects the manner and degree of openness that group members can begin to express toward each other and to each of the therapists. Openness in the co-therapy team lays the foundation for a group atmosphere that is facilitative of free and candid emotional and cognitive exchanges and a low level of defensiveness.

On a group level, a lack of openness may lead to a defensive structure whereby co-leaders present either a united front in which they deny differences or oppositional styles in which they deny similarities. Whether this is done overtly or covertly, it will sabotage the group by distracting energy toward the co-therapy relationship. Defensive operations will be stimulated in the group-as-a-whole, leading to splitting and subgrouping that will hinder the group's development.

*Issue 4. Negotiation:* The degree of clarity that co-leaders achieve in their contract affects the amount of time clients spend absorbed in covert conflicts between therapists. Lack of clarity contributes to the clients' confusions regarding the therapeutic contract that they themselves are entering.

On a group level the lack of clarity in the contract between co-leaders may arouse confusion in the members regarding their roles in helping the group to proceed in a clear and helpful way. Group members quickly size up the tasks performed by each of the co-leaders and any differences in power. They also notice the degree to which these are resolved comfortably. This becomes a model to the group members for the management of their own roles and differences.

## PHASE 1 Co-Therapist/Group Issues: Implications for Clients and Group-as-a-Whole

*Issue 5. Compatibility:* It is a very important aspect of any Task Leader's role to give clear guidelines to a group about how to get the job done for which they have gathered. When this role is shared equally, it becomes extremely important that co-therapists present a coherent image of what therapy is about and how it is to proceed. They are susceptible to being perceived in oppositional ways by clients who are already involved in splitting or other defensive mechanisms. If the co-therapists have not taken the time to deal with their differences, in fact, even to formulate an umbrella concept that holds their discrepant views together, then there is a great risk that clients'projections and fixations will remain unexplored and unresolved.

Since all groups present a complexity of data to be addressed, there is always a question about which issues to address and when and how to address them. The more compatible the orientation of the therapists, the more likely they will be to approach group-level problems by striving for the same goals and agreeing on the hierarchy of the issues to be addressed.

*Issue 6. Bonding:* Agreement about how clients are to be shared determines how available the therapists will be to clients in the group, and therefore such agreement determines the nature of the bonds that clients can form with each of the co-leaders. It is important for clients in the group to feel free to bond with both leaders and to have the opportunity to explore the differences between those bonds. Bonding has implications for the kinds of issues, conflicts, and developmental blocks on which clients are able to work in the group. In order for this work to be accomplished, the two leaders must be open to client involvement with both of them. They must also have an open communication process for dealing with the issues that are raised for clients by the complexity of bonding with two therapists.

Flexible bonding of clients to either co-therapist may enhance the clients' openness about their needs and preferences, making it easier to see their issues clearly in the group. The leaders must be clear about what is acceptable bonding. If they are not clear, unexplored or unresolved differences between the formal, explicit rules and their informal expectations may lead to burying important issues in the group or even to stimulating acting-out by clients.

*Issue 7. Stresses:* The degree to which co-therapists process their own stress and therefore understand each other more fully determines the clarity with which they approach clients and their issues. Transference and countertransference are often stimulated when therapists are under stress and behave in an atypical manner. The degree to which therapists understand the context of the stress that affects each of them allows them to differentiate clients' projections from reality more fully.

The way in which co-leaders manage the stresses they experience is probably the most overtly observable aspect of their collaboration or lack thereof. This becomes a model to the group members of identifying, discussing, and problem solving the stresses that the group's composite conflicts will create.

The evolution of the co-therapy relationship will either be facilitated or hindered by certain organizational norms and attitudes. Reciprocally, the development of a new relationship between two members of a professional staff has impacts upon the organization within which they function. In the next section we will discuss these matters in the context of the same seven issues presented above.

### PHASE 1 Dyadic Relationship Issues: Implications for the Institution or Group Private Practice

*Issues 1 and 2. Attraction and Gains:* Because of the press of demands on institutions or group private practices (when the practice is large and has a hierarchical structure), it is often a low priority for them to consider the needs and interests of the persons involved when selecting co-therapists. It is quite possible that management may not understand the implications of its decisions in co-therapist selection in terms of how such decisions will affect the quality of the delivery of services to patients in the group or the morale of the staff. Nevertheless, the institution or private practice creates conditions that determine whether or not staff will address the interpersonal concerns that affect their abilities in the delivery of services. At the most basic level, staff commitment to the group they will lead and to the organization itself is greatly influenced by policies regarding staff involvement in decision making about assignments. Arbitrary assignments generate a poor level of involvement.

*Issue 3. Communication:* In order for staff to achieve an open and nondefensive way of communicating, an institution or group private practice needs to facilitate openness about role and status differences between the various professional disciplines within the organization. These differences are often connected with varying interests, concerns, and responsibilities in the context of working together on cases. This will strongly affect the degree to which professionals are able to use their talents and to learn from each other.The alternative generally leads to the dissipation of energy in nonproductive, competitive behavior.

Openness across disciplines within the organization in the context of co-therapy usually results in maximum feedback ultimately to the organization itself. The co-therapy consultation process tends to uncover or clarify problems in the organizational context of the group and in its policies as these impact the clients and the staff and the conduct of the group.

*Issue 4. Negotiation:* The clearer the contract that co-therapists have with each other and with their institution or group private practice, the less likely it is that these systems will adversely affect each other or the delivery of services in the therapy group. In fact, the creation of a clear interpersonal contract between co-therapists depends on a clear contract with the organization as well. The latter contract not only defines the parameters of the group but should also define the authority of the leaders and especially the limits of their authority. In most settings this is accomplished through discussion with the supervisor or administrator or both.

*PHASE 1 Co-Therapist–Group Issues: Implications for the Institution or Group Private Practice*

*Issue 5. Compatibility:* The institution or group private practice holds the primary responsibility for setting norms concerning treatment philosophy, types of interventions, and the dominant aspects of style of therapist behavior. This provides an umbrella that facilitates co-leaders in having a dialogue with each other as they develop treatment strategies consistent with the overall aims of the organization. In addition, if the co-therapists feel able to address or influence changes in treatment approaches that lead to better patient outcome, this will greatly affect their professional image and confidence level as a team. Further, the clients' perceptions of an organization are largely mediated through their perception of staff competence, effectiveness, and professionalism.

*Issue 6. Bonding:* Organizational norms about ownership of clients strongly influence the stance of the co-therapy team in regard to sharing responsibility in their work with clients. The degree to which clients are shared by co-leaders affects the amount of dialogue and consultation that goes on between them and with supervisors and other professionals involved with the case. When co-leaders can openly discuss their relationships with clients, they influence the norms in the direction of openness for all levels of an organization to examine their own relationships with clients.

*Issue 7. Stresses:* Stress created by the agency is among the issues to be dealt with by co-leaders. It is best when each one is free to discuss his or her own relationship to the agency with the co-leader and the supervisor and to develop a supportive, noncompetitive stance in these discussions. Stress between co-leaders impacts on the organization also, affecting their relationships in other contexts than just the group. Co-leaders need to discuss the implications of their collaboration with respect to their differing roles in the organization, and their colleagues in the organization need to be free to discuss how the partnership affects them.

Co-therapists who have chosen to work together and are in a private practice that is small and without a hierarchical structure still must address their expectations and their interest in each other as they plan to co-lead. Our view is that relationship building or rebuilding occurs whenever there is a new task. In an existing relationship it is important to attend to the basic issues outlined in this first phase vis-á-vis the task at hand. Most of what has been outlined earlier about Phase 1 applies to the independent practice team as well. Although they may not be in an organization, they probably have a relationshp that goes beyond the particular group they will be co-leading. As this contract becomes defined, it will probably have implications for other aspects of their personal and professional relationship. At each phase it will be important to address those implications and to keep this work clearly differentiated from other tasks.

### Guidelines for Institutions or Group Private Practices Regarding Co-Therapy

It is important for organizations to be clear about what they expect from their group therapy program. If there are minimal or even unclear expectations about the purpose and importance of their group therapy program, then there is usually little investment by the co-leaders in this complex process or it may even become impossible for them to structure an effective working relationship.

Often, however, organizations highly value group therapy and have a well-thought-out system for organizing patients into the kind of groups that they need. The failures usually come from not realizing that there is an equally important process involved in the selection of staff members to be co-leaders and in not structuring a process that will insure the development of an effective work team.

The following are some ideas that may be helpful to institutions or group private practices interested in setting up or improving an existing group therapy program.

1. When possible, allow staff members to have some choice of co-therapy partners. Then, encourage them to be clear with each other about their personal and professional expectations and goals.

2. Allow teams to work together long enough to be able to develop their working relationship sufficiently to be an effective team, that is to at least reach Phase 3 in their relationship building.

3. If the time that the co-therapists have to work together is shorter than the length of stay of the group members, then it is important that one leader remain in the group in an on-going way to create continuity for the clients and the group process. It is important to define clearly and narrowly the group's purpose and to define realistically the roles of the two leaders because they will not have equal influence as Task Leaders of the group. Although equal in other respects as co-therapists, practically speaking, the short-term partner should have limited functions compared to the long-term partner. Finally, it is important to share this information with the clients.

4. Where leaders are in training as either nequipos or co-learners, the time of their participation in a long-term group may vary also. In these cases, the long-term partner would be either the supervisor or the co-learner who has served more hours with the group. The institution or group private practice must limit their expectations of what the short-term partner can accomplish and must establish ways to measure the progress of the trainees without unfair comparison with their supervisor or co-learner with greater seniority. Once again the group members must be informed of the different functions they can expect their leaders to perform.

5. Give a high priority to conceptual compatibility when selecting co-leaders who will have short-term contact. If they will have long-term contact as co-leaders, then time must be devoted to consultation not only about the clients but about the co-leaders' relationship and the coordination of their orientations.

6. Formulate guidelines concerning the sharing of clients, both in and out of the group therapy setting. This may be less of a concern in inpatient systems that have a team approach to patients already.

7. Encourage an open system of communication between leaders, especially in the supervisory context, so that their feelings and reactions to each other and to the patients can be shared.

8. Insure a system of supervision for all co-leaders in which the expectation is explicit that there will be consultation time with each other and with a supervisor or facilitator (even experienced co-leaders benefit from special attention at the start of a new co-leadership relationship and supervision provides this). When co-leaders have a forum where they can talk with a supervisor, the likelihood that they will address their issues is increased dramatically. In those instances where the senior co-leader is also the supervisor (see Chapter 2), the focus during consultation is usually not on the co-therapy relationship. It is harder under these conditions for the two parties to negotiate their feelings and ideas as partners in the co-therapy venture. This is an inherent difficulty and challenge for the nequipo team

## PHASE 2: FORMING AN IDENTITY

Phase 2 involves forming the structure and identity of the co-therapy team. The co-therapists must formulate norms and guidelines, develop methods for coordinating their efforts, and devise strategies for coping with stress. They must also define goals to which they can both make a commitment as they establish a working relationship. A struggle ensues in which the co-leaders compete for dominance, influence, and/or power as a way to achieve a feeling of comfort. It is natural that irritations and aggressions will arise and may seem very personal in their origin; yet, they are usually the result of misunderstandings as the co-leaders struggle to define their partnership. This phase challenges the therapists' skills in identification of issues, clarification of feelings, and negotiation of solutions. This is a phase that leads either to the formation of an emerging identity for the team or to the dissolution of the co-leadership arrangement. Co-leaders who get stuck in a competitive process should not continue to attempt to co-lead a group. The general recommendation is to spend a good deal of time during this phase discussing issues and resolving differences in order to move through it as efficiently as possible. Below we outline the seven issues (already discussed) as they are expressed in Phase 2 of the emerging co-therapy relationship.

## The Seven Issues as Expressed in Phase 2

*PHASE 2 Dyadic Relationship Issues*

*Issue 1. Attraction:* The strength of interest and attraction the co-leaders have for each other is potentially an important motivational factor in helping them work through a natural desire to dominate and compete at this phase in their relationship. It is typical that narcissistic issues emerge at this point. Leaders are trying to demonstrate their knowledge and expertise, and each one may find the other one's style irritating, "wrong," or not understandable at times. Depending on the power of these narcissistic, competitive issues and the degree of personalizing, co-leaders need to have a comparable desire to get to know and respect each other as different and separate individuals. In addition, the tension of forming an identity as a team needs to be viewed as coming from a natural struggle at this phase that occurs independently of personality characteristics and professional differences.

*Issue 2. Gains:* For Phase 2 to be resolved efficiently, each therapist must view the relationship as having the potential to increase respect for abilities as well as providing acceptance for limitations. The extent to which they get to know themselves and each other better determines how fully and openly each therapist will participate in the co-therapy relationship and in the group. They must avoid seeking self-esteem at each other's expense.

*Issue 3. Communication:* It takes special effort and tolerance of ambiguity to communicate in an open, nondefensive manner. A mature processing of issues can create an atmosphere of stimulation and exploration. If, however, their discussions generate threat, there may be a tendency for co-leaders to resort to primitive patterns of defensiveness that foster one-upmanship and stereotyping. The degree to which defensiveness predominates will determine whether or not the therapists will be able to engage in a process of listening to each other in an open, noncompetitive manner.

*Issue 4. Negotiation:* Co-leaders need clearly to differentiate their contract from other work or personal relationship issues. This becomes particularly important in this phase because role relationships vis-á-vis other tasks or in other contexts may confuse the co-therapy communication process. These overlapping roles and issues must be sorted out and differentiated if the co-therapy relationship is to be clear and understandable. In particular, the co-therapists must explore the implications of power and authority differences between them outside of the group in order to facilitate their working relationship in the group.

When these issues are not addressed, any problem or discomfort in their out-of-group relationship will tend to influence or even be acted out in the group. The potential to confuse and act out feelings from one area of involvement to another becomes more tempting at this particular phase. Discrepancies in perceived power or injury incurred in their out-of-group relationship are especially difficult issues for the co-therapy relationship in the group. The resolution of Phase 2 depends on the clarification of important differences and the achievement of a mutually agreed-on style for handling them.

## PHASE 2 Co-Therapist–Group Issues

*Issue 5. Compatibility:* Being able to engage in an open and nondefensive style of communication becomes essential if the co-therapists are to be able to understand emerging differences and similarities in their theoretical orientations, in their preferred intervention strategies and in their styles of interaction. Differences between the way co-leaders described their orientations during the contracting phase and the way they actually interact in group begin to become more evident. A commitment to process the confusion this causes and to negotiate differences to the point of resolution becomes critical if a deeper understanding about their modes of working is to be achieved.

The differences identified could be too great for collaborative effort to continue, and the co-leadership relationship may need to end. In this case a commitment to a constructive termination process and discussion is necessary if hurt feelings are to be minimized. Also, the implications for the group need to be processed and handled in unison so as to prevent damaging experiences to clients.

*Issue 6. Bonding:* The natural push–pull of Phase 2 makes this issue the most difficult to handle well. Client–therapist bonds are usually important to all therapists. Those who have experience with team efforts will find this period easier to handle. Those who have no experience with team efforts will probably struggle both internally and interpersonally during this time. In either case, sharing their experience will significantly deepen the relationship between co-leaders and will lay the foundation for a collaboratively developed style for their work in the future. There are many forces that can impede this positive outcome. There is a natural, almost seductive tendency for therapists to want to be liked or admired by group members. Co-leaders may have a difficult time acknowledging, exploring, and owning these feelings in an open manner. When they are unable to do that, in-group competing can potentially divide group members into subgroups based on loyalty to one or the other of the co-therapists.

*Issue 7. Stresses:* The co-therapy team generates stress, and it is multiplied by the stresses the group places on the team. This norm-generating phase can be enormously draining if a defensive style of communication gets set in motion and causes injuries to self-esteem. This may be deliberately caused or can occur inadvertently. If co-leaders have support to help them sort out their differences and to learn accurately about each other during this time, there will be a significant lowering of their anxiety and tension. When the co-therapists cope successfully with the stresses in their team and in the group, they facilitate the evolution of a supportive relationship and generate data for working on personal and professional growth. The main focus of this phase is the creation of a structure for the co-therapist team. This means clarifying norms and goals, generating rules of operation, exploring differences and similarities, and defining roles. When the energy of the co-leaders stays clearly on these issues Phase 2 is bridged efficiently, and stress is kept to a minimum.

## PHASE 2 Dyadic Relationship Issues: Implications for Clients and Group-as-a-Whole

*Issue 1. Attraction:* It is difficult to hide the strain that co-therapists experience during this period even if the partners relate in a relatively relaxed or even humorous manner. When we hear things we like, the natural concomitants of the process of getting to know another person are feelings of excitement, delight, or warmth. When we hear things we don't like or don't understand, we tend to become irritated, to back off, or to experience doubt. This advance/retreat characteristic is typical of this phase. When co-leaders recognize that this is natural and devote sufficient time to dialogue and resolve differences, they will model an important process to the group, that is, how to build a healthy relationship. On the other hand, when co-leaders are perceived as competitive in a one-upmanship manner, clients will be less likely to risk sharing vulnerable material.

On a group level, the co-leaders' competitive style may become a model for the way members will handle comparable interpersonal issues.

*Issue 2. Gains:* The co-leaders model the future norms of the group as they work out and balance their relationship with one another. As clients view co-leaders either struggling or negotiating with each other, they may develop concerns about their own needs being met. It is natural that some insecurity could be expressed in the group during the therapists' Phase 2 process. Co-leaders in their dyad and in the group-as-a-whole must develop norms about how they will handle the needs of each person. The important issue here is whether a sensitivity develops for each person's struggles and a genuine concern is generated to address them.

*Issue 3. Communication:* An atmosphere of mutual exploration between co-leaders stimulates clients to be exploratory in the group as well. Seeing co-therapists handle their own competitiveness and limitations in a constructive and efficient manner tends to create hope in the group that their own issues with each other can also be dealt with effectively. Behaviorally, the co-therapists present the clients with an alternative to their own regressive models for coping. If, however, co-therapists become ensnarled in a defensive pattern that is characterized by either intense emotions or a protracted, submerged struggle, they will create an atmosphere in which clients will express regressive behavior. Intrapsychically, the co-therapists would reinforce the effect of whatever dysfunctional relationship contributed to their clients' emotional problems in the first place. A sense of hopelessness is stimulated in certain clients and symptomotology is increased.

Therapists need to have a sensitive awareness of the way their defensive styles may impact or even damage the group-level processing. A power struggle between therapists will tend to create subgrouping and an "Us" versus "Them" atmosphere. Emerging group-structural issues will not get processed, and the group may develop norms centered around manipulation and competition.

*Issue 4. Negotiation:* When co-leaders have been able to differentiate their co-therapy relationship from other areas in which their lives overlap, they have more energy available to focus on encountering clients in a powerful way in the group with each other's help and support. When they are subtly playing out inequalities and stressful issues from other aspects of their relationship, they will tend to function independently from each other. They will not collaborate or support each other in encountering clients or be as effective in engaging the rest of the group in the work of any particular member.

The management of issues of the group-as-a-whole generally requires a co-therapy team that is able to collaborate. Group-as-a-whole phenomena are often complex and difficult to identify when the group is in process. Co-leaders who freely offer their observations, feelings, confusions, and hypotheses to each other and can analyze and develop strategies together are more likely to understand the major as well as the subtle, minor themes in a group.

*PHASE 2 Co-Therapist–Group Issues: Implications for the Clients and Group-as-a-Whole*

*Issue 5. Compatibility:* Differences in orientation may stimulate discussions about clients in which differing sets of data become available to generate new insights, giving the clients a richer resource. The danger, however, is that these discussions may lead to impasses about case management. Co-therapists may experience competitive feelings with each other as they differentially respond to clients. If this is acted out in the group, a variety of consequences may occur: For example, each therapist may develop his own theme with clients, or the two therapists may actually undercut or contradict each other's interventions. These consequences lead to a threatening environment for clients and may cause them to disengage or even to experience some damage.

On the group-as-a-whole level, if therapists are able to collaborate in the face of their different points of view, they will facilitate norms that allow the use of the whole range of feelings and ideas in the group members. If the therapists are split in their views of either how to conduct the group or how to work with individual clients, then the group-as-a-whole will reach an impasse in the development of norms regarding the way they all work together therapeutically. It is then likely that the group will get stuck in its own Phase II (see Table A of the Appendix).

*Issue 6. Bonding:* The primary implication of the bonding issue for the clients is whether or not therapists show support and involvement in the clients' emerging issues. Therapists who are actively addressing their own issues during their Phase 2 process will present an even and calm emotional position to clients. Clients in turn will interpret this as stability and will respond by investing in their own work in the group. If therapists do not work together, various splits will emerge as the clients align with one of the leaders. In a competitive process there is a tendency for therapists to act out in a way that encourages these splits, using them for their own ends. The danger here is that they are potentially recreating the kind of dysfunctional family system that caused the clients' problems in the first place. The ability of therapists to support each other during this time is critical. Clients should be free to rely on both co-leaders to help them work through their developmental impasses.

*Issue 7. Stresses:* The level of stress and the degree to which it is managed competently is the issue that has the most immediate and direct impact on clients. Since co-leaders who are in the second phase of co-therapy development are probably in a group that is in an early phase as well, the clients are looking to the therapists for guidance and intervention to help them process similar issues in the group. Therapists who are managing their own interpersonal stresses will be much more available to help the clients process group events such as competition.

## PHASE 2 Dyadic Relationship Issues: Implications for the Institution or Group Private Practice

*Issue 1. Attraction:* Agencies may take advantage of co-therapists' differences for their own ends, exacerbating the problems and blocking resolutions or they may take a mature position through the supervisory process to resolve problems and facilitate growth of staff members. Fellow staff may take a systems or developmental point of view toward co-therapists in conflict or may take sides based on personalities and personal alliances. Co-therapists themselves may take their relationship problems and escalate them into staff problems, or they may seek supervisory help in their resolution, taking the opportunity to differentiate further the co-therapy relationship from other staff involvements.

*Issue 2. Gains:* The organization itself has a set of values and policies that will strongly determine the potential for viewing a co-therapy relationship as an opportunity for growth and development for the participants. One direct way this is expressed is by the amount of time devoted to supervision or consultation. This is an expensive investment and usually only pays off for an organization if they retain mature staff members or establish the organization as a quality training center.

*Issue 3. Communication:* The organization can create a powerful set of norms that reinforce accuracy and openness in communication. In this kind of atmosphere, anxiety and defensiveness will be reduced and consultation will be sought for problems that are not easily resolved. In organizations that are themselves caught in competitive dynamics, Phase 2 tensions between co-therapists can easily escalate by being related in some way to the broader organizational issues. The goal of a healthy organization should be to create an atmosphere in which interpersonal and structural problems are openly addressed at all levels: the dyad, the administrative unit, and the organization as a whole.

*Issue 4. Negotiation:* Some organizations maintain rigid lines of differentiation between professional discipline and/or administrative units. An organization has to be willing to address the implications of their policies and to allow staff members of different status or positions to establish a co-therapy relationship based on equal responsibility. This will greatly facilitate co-leaders in establishing a sense of clarity about how their power and knowledge can be used in their therapy group.

### PHASE 2 Co-Therapist Group Issues: Implications for Institutions or Group Private Practice

*Issue 5. Compatibility:* The organization itself and the supervisory personnel in particular need to be clear about their own policies and orientation in the conduct of group work. Without this clarity they will add one more component of confusion to the process of the co-therapists during Phase 2. Lack of clarity will also add to the competition. Co-therapy teams caught in Phase 2 require strong, fair refereeing from a supervisor who is committed to assist co-leaders in developing honest, respectful communication with each other.

*Issue 6. Bonding:* Organizational policy regarding formal responsibility for the sharing of clients is essential. Any discrepancies in how boundaries are set for therapists in their interaction with clients will generate confusion and misunderstandings and may lead to acting out. Both therapists and clients need to be clear about the organizational policy and the group rules regarding client–therapist involvement. It is an important norm in all supervisory processes that the potential healing power in the client-to-therapist bonding process be understood and maximally utilized.

*Issue 7. Stresses:* It is important for the organization to have policies and procedures for addressing stress-producing events in therapists' lives, whether these originate inside or outside of the organization, and to provide active help. When co-therapists are under stress from events outside of the work context, and they are occupied with the significant structural issues of their relationship, there is less energy available to sort out what is happening internally and in the group.

### PHASE 3 BUILDING A TEAM

When co-leaders have sufficiently sorted out their structural issues and formulated their goals, they begin to communicate in a more open and specific manner. The co-therapists begin to develop an operational model for handling the various issues that arise between themselves, with their clients, and with the group. They experiment with ways to cope with changes in their work setting or personal lives. They also

begin to work out a style for their co-leadership in which they coordinate both communication and intervention differences. This may
involve some differentiation of leadership function in the group.

### The Seven Issues as Expressed in Phase 3

*PHASE 3 Dyadic Relationship Issues*

*Issue 1. Attraction:* The interest and attraction of the co-leaders toward one another helps propel them in the direction of providing
support to each other and of generating cooperation. As a result, trust
begins to be operationally defined. To achieve this trust-building
process, any leftover feelings and issues from the previous phase are
resolved, and any damaging experiences that may have occurred are
further repaired. This work generally frees energy for the positive
aspects of the relationship to emerge and for investment in the group.
The co-leaders begin to develop tolerance, understanding, and sensitivity for each other. Their efforts become focused on learning to
appreciate each other's unique style, contributions and actions. Failure
to explore openly leftover feelings and concerns from the previous
phases results in compartmentalizing unfinished business, freezing
energy, and blocking investment in the relationship and in the group.
The residual effect would be either to limit the range of activity and
emotion within which the relationship is conducted or to prevent
continued evolution to later phases.

*Issue 2. Gains:* A peer consultation relationship develops when co-
leaders help one another with their concerns about the group. There is
a movement toward the co-therapy relationship being used as a source
for personal and professional growth. Collaboration in the context of
consultation stimulates an openness to explore new perceptions of self,
of others, and of the group. This leads the co-therapists to an activation
of their potential as therapeutic agents and as resources to each other
for new learning. When co-leaders are unable to explore the personal
and professional dimensions of their relationship, it can become rigid
and noncollaborative. Under such circumstances, the co-therapists
may be unable to process new information adequately.

*Issue 3. Communication:* Communication difficulties usually arise
from actual differences of viewpoint rather than from defensive patterns based on interpersonal projections and competition. As a result of
an increased sense of trust and respect, the co-leaders actually begin to
know each other as distinct individuals. Differences of opinion become
vehicles for the partners to become better acquainted with each other's

perspectives. The projections of Phase 2 can now lead to self-reflection. The communication themes in this phase are listening, cooperating, and understanding rather than focusing on winning or losing. Failure to achieve this level of openness results in stopping the exchange of new information between co-leaders and limits the potential that a coherent therapeutic style would develop.

*Issue 4. Negotiation:* The clearer picture of the co-therapists as individuals that emerges in this phase leads to a reality-based identity as a team. Prior to Phase 3 leaders seldom operate as a team. Instead, they tend to work in a parallel or even competitive fashion. Co-leaders need to make a more positive commitment to the co-therapy bond and the establishment of a collaborative style as a team. Emotionally, they begin to develop a sense of cohesion and anticipation. In operational terms, the co-therapists begin to develop an exploratory attitude toward the understanding and use of their strengths and limitations as they interact with each other and the group.

## PHASE 3 Co-Therapist–Group Issues

*Issue 5. Compatibility:* The co-therapists are now productively beginning to negotiate therapeutic strategies that incorporate their differing styles and orientations. A therapeutic identity is emerging that encompasses assets and takes into account the limitations of the two leaders. Both long-term strategies and short-term interventions for problems and crises that arise in the group are becoming operationalized. In the context of specific planning for individual clients and for the management of the group-as-a-whole, the co-therapists are planning the ways they will use their talents and skills efficiently and in coordination with each other. When differences in the styles of the co-leaders are not used collaboratively, rigid boundaries will develop that limit the creativity of their interventions and the comfort of their work.

*Issue 6. Bonding:* Phase 3 provides an opportunity for co-leaders to share clients in a collaborative manner. The co-leaders begin to appreciate their unique and different contributions to clients and respect each other's skills. This lays the groundwork for a flexible system to develop, facilitating the evolution of the bonding of clients to co-leaders in a complex process. Some co-leaders allow clients to switch from one leader to another for individual work, depending on the developmental issues the clients are working through. Others believe it is important to maintain the same therapist throughout for individual work. Although it seems to be rare at this time, some groups do not include the option for individual therapy. In any case, this phase creates the opportunity to develop the patterns that will work best for the co-leaders and for the group members. The question of bonding can also become the arena for more submerged competitive issues to arise, especially around letting go of ownership of clients. In a less defensive and more collaborative atmosphere this competition can be managed productively, leading to a set of policies that meet the needs of both leaders and clients.

*Issue 7. Stresses:* As Phase 3 begins any leftover confusion or anxiety from Phase 2 may need to be acknowledged and worked through. The stresses that are specific to Phase 3 are centered around working through any misunderstandings that come up as co-leaders make a serious effort to develop a collaborative relationship. By talking about their misunderstandings, most co-therapists reduce their stress and redirect their energy to the examination of group and individual dynamics.

## PHASE 3 Dyadic Relationship Issues: Implications for Clients and Group-as-a-Whole

*Issue 1. Attraction:* When the group members experience the co-leaders as collaborative, they express an increased willingness to bring up and work on material in a more focused manner. The group members can sense a more open and cooperative relationship between co-leaders who create a sense of safety in the group and a model for cooperation with each other as they address their mutual tasks. When co-leaders are able to trust each other and are less embroiled in power struggles, they become more able to identify structural problems that emerge in the group-as-a-whole. In addition, the co-leaders can more easily identify their own impasses and the various ways these may parallel group-level impasses.

*Issue 2. Gains:* Therapists who are operationally trusting tend to give each other more latitude and support in pursuing hunches and intuitions about individual clients. They begin to let each other take risks in engaging the deeper meaning of clients' behavior in the group. As clients sense this change in atmosphere, they become less defensive and more willing to disclose themselves at a deeper level.

As co-leaders operate in a more cooperative manner concerning their own needs, there is a greater likelihood that group-level themes will be addressed. Otherwise, these themes if unaddressed will inter-fere with group members' self exploration and with group-as-a-whole development.

*Issue 3. Communication:* As the co-therapists communicate more openly, they will employ more effective interventions and strategies for individual clients. When therapists feel free to share their ideas and observations in a spontaneous manner, more data are generated, leading to a greater understanding of clients. The team becomes a model to clients on how to interact nondefensively as co-leaders begin to communicate more openly with each other in the group. When co-leaders feel free to disagree with each other in a nonjudgmental manner, it helps create norms in the group that allow each person to express a wider range of feelings and associations.

On a group level, the potential for greater acceptance for diversity emerges and, therefore, a greater acceptance of the clients as they are at the moment. The facilitation of a nonjudgmental atmosphere models for the clients the hope that interpersonal relationships can lead to positive growth. They learn that systems can develop conditions that lead to different outcomes than those taught them by their prior experiences in life.

*Issue 4. Negotiation:* As the co-therapists are able to sort out the complexity in their own struggle to work together, they become more able to focus on the work of facilitating each client. This allows a greater use of all the data being generated by the clients and increases the likelihood that the co-leaders will have a deeper and more complex understanding of each client. As the co-leaders develop a clear, consis-tent, and identifiable style, clients have more of a sense of how to ask for help and how to utilize help in the group context.

Both the co-therapy team and the group must develop their own identities. It is virtually impossible for a group to become a team with its own characteristics and traditions when its therapists do not have their own. Moreover, groups over time present increasingly more complicated issues for resolution and require co-leaders who are able to adapt and change rapidly. Not unlike a football team whose coach must be able to read the changes in his players and in the team's ability to function optimally, the co-leaders must be able to adapt to the emerging developmental issues of the group and of the members. Phase 3 is a time when the co-leaders develop a sense of being together and of relying on each other's strengths. This is necessary for group-level tasks to be clarified and negotiated effectively.

*PHASE 3 Co-Therapist–Group Issues: Implications for Clients and Group-as-a-Whole*

*Issue 5. Compatibility:* As co-therapists are able to utilize each others' intuitions, clinical judgments, and theoretical orientations in a more cooperative manner, a richer and more complex picture of the client's behavior emerges. This provides a chance for the clients to develop a better understanding of their problems and to find resources in the group to resolve them.

At the group-as-a-whole level, the group can now incorporate as norms a wider range of the therapist's therapeutic skills. This means the group can work through problems at the individual and group structural levels. Clients can begin to take risks in helping one another when they see their therapists open to a range of insights and styles. The therapeutic power of a group is the result of the collaboration of the therapeutic skills of all of its members and leaders.

*Issue 6. Bonding:* When therapists present a clear and flexible picture of how clients are shared, the implications for the treatment of the individual member is profound. The emergence of transference and the reenactment of developmental impasses can be more effectively addressed as clients feel free to utilize both of the therapists. Often it was the rigidity in the original parental system that led to developmental fixation. When co-leaders are able to discuss openly the powerful ways in which clients want different expressions of love from each therapist, the clients are able to verbalize their needs, to feel understood, and to have their feelings acknowledged. This validation is often an essential step for clients because they can come to understand their own feelings and impulses in the context of the general human condition and not as aberrations.

On a group level norms are evolving that allow clients to acknowledge their bonds to the therapists and to each other and to use this material as a therapeutic focus. These norms permit the group to acknowledge the significance of each relationship and encourage opportunity for discussion and exploration with the support of the group-as-a-whole.

*Issue 7. Stresses:* As co-therapists are able to form a more trusting, collaborative, and exploratory relationship, they can examine the way the therapy group affects them and is affected by them. Discrepancies, differences, and similarities between the co-therapists and the group members regarding the therapy process and the progress of the group can be clarified, and their implications can be examined. Openness in exploring interactional aspects of systems lays the groundwork for viewing the complexity of the change process at multiple levels.

### PHASE 3 Dyadic Relationship Issues: Implications for the Institution or Group Private Practice

*Issues 1 and 2. Attraction and Gains:* On the institutional or group private practice level, co-leaders who are operationally becoming more trusting of each other are more likely to be comfortable sharing their experiences with other staff. In addition, co-leaders are more likely to benefit from the input of others. When co-leaders are more trusting and appear to be gaining in a personal and professional way, there is a natural tendency for other staff members to see more clearly the value of a noncompetitive, collaborative work style. More positive, cooperative work norms in the system can be strengthened since co-leaders may be less willing to engage in power struggles and manipulations that lead to defensive, nonproductive interactions on the organizational level. On the other hand, when the organization is caught in a destructive, competitive, or scapegoating style of operation, the co-therapy relationship can become a safe place to process the tensions and find constructive strategies. However, the co-therapy relationship has just entered a productive phase and is still vulnerable to outside pressures. The ability of the organization to support and model the value of a cooperative and trusting professional work style will facilitate and strengthen the co-leaders' attempts to create such a relationship.

*Issue 3. Communication:* When a nondefensive style of communication is valued in an organization, co-leaders are more likely to address systemic problems in the work setting. If the organization's policy is positive about group therapy, yet operationally the organization undermines the norms required to facilitate effective co-leadership and group development, a nondefensive atmosphere will help the co-therapists point out the contradictions. On the other hand, when a supervisor's insights can be heard in an open manner as he or she represents the organization's viewpoint, co-leaders are more likely to see how their attitudes may be undermining goals and objectives of the organization. If there are true differences between systems that are not reconcilable, then there is an opportunity to negotiate an ending of either the group or the co-therapy relationship in a mutually respectful manner.

*Issue 4. Negotiation:* For co-therapists to clarify effectively and strengthen their emerging identity, they require protection as they begin to define the needs of the group and themselves as leaders. The co-leaders require active support in articulating who they are. As their partnership becomes more visible, and a stronger commitment to their tasks and goals becomes operational, the organization benefits from their collaboration.

*PHASE 3 Co-Therapist/Group Issues: Implications for the Institution or Group Private Practice*

*Issue 5. Compatibility:* The supervisor's interventions should help to clarify the substantive therapeutic issues in both the co-leadership and the case-management aspects of the work. It is important to help the co-leaders shift from discussing their issues as personality problems to seeing the genuine differences in their thinking and in their responses to client and group issues. When fellow staff begin to communicate in this stimulating and cooperative manner about cases they share, there is a tendency to apply a similar style to other aspects of their work, thus improving the work atmosphere of the organization in general. In addition, the underlying therapeutic philosophy of an organization is often not clearly articulated, nor are the discrepancies in theory and practice clearly labeled. It is often the case that when co-leaders are able to clarify the assumptions that underlie their therapeutic interventions, they are also able to identify comparable assumptions in all the various systems of the organization.

*Issue 6. Bonding:* For co-leaders to build a therapeutic identity effectively they must establish a clear and cooperative approach to sharing clients that is congruent with the organization's goals and role expectations. The supervisor should facilitate and encourage the sharing of clients and a collaborative style of intervention. Each therapist performs the functions he or she can do most effectively with each client at any time. This style contributes to an atmosphere of consultation and collaboration on cases in the organization. Its policies should allow and encourgage this.

*Issue 7. Stresses:* As co-leaders establish a more cooperative work style, they are better able to name the various stresses that impinge on their relationship and to help each other find better coping strategies. What the co-therapists learn is passed along to the organization saving time and effort for the entire staff.

## CONCLUSIONS

The focus in this chapter has been on the evolution of the co-therapy relationship of leaders with relatively equal experience in conducting therapy groups. Co-therapists may differ in terms of their experience or knowledge, and each of these differences will have its own set of consequences for the informal and formal structure of the co-therapy relationship and for the group. We know from our own research on groups that if the leaders possess unequal experience with groups, the clients will not perceive them both as Task Leaders in the group even though both leaders make meaningful therapeutic interventions (Beck & Peters, 1981; Beck et al., 1989). This is especially true when students, interns, or residents are co-leading with staff therapists or with their professors (nequipos). Such arrangements have implications for the supervisory or consultation processes. The planning of interventions in the group must take this factor into account. Our process research also shows that the student member of a nequipo team does not speak as much in a group as the four emergent leaders (including the Task Leader). This indicates a hesitancy to venture forth but also a recognition that the role is different from the Task Leader's.

We have elaborated in some detail because we assumed we were writing for therapists who want to commit to on-going co-therapy relationships. We also assumed an involvement with relatively long-term groups devoted to intensive psychotherapy, where the quality of the relationship would make a significant difference over time and throughout the course of the group's life. We are aware that many groups are short-term or narrower in their task focus than the groups assumed above. In these instances it is still important to address the issues outlined in the chapter. However, we recognize that some leaders will not want to invest so much time or explore to such depth as we have described. Short-term groups and inpatient groups create built-in pressures on the co-leaders to move their own processes along as quickly as possible so that they will be able to make the necessary interventions when they are needed by clients in the group. In these instances, it is especially important to manage differences between leaders in a direct, explicit, and reasonably objective manner so as to prevent confusion and frustration in the group members and problems in the structural formation of the group.

We have presented the first three phases of a nine-phase theory for the development of a co-therapy relationship. This theory represents our initial attempt to describe the development of the informal aspects of the co-therapy relationship. Each phase has a major developmental task to address. This task is examined from two perspectives: first, we outline the dyadic relationship issues that define the parameters of interpersonal evolution; second, we outline the co-therapist–group issues that address how co-leaders will coordinate with each other to handle the various tasks that are necessary in the treatment of clients in the context of a group. We come from a systems-theory perspective that emphasizes the isomorphic processes among the individual system, co-leadership system, group-as-a-whole system, and the organization or group private practice system. In particular, we believe that groups do not achieve a higher level of phase development than the one the co-therapists have achieved in their own relationship.

The model suggests that therapists should address in an explicit manner their interests in and attractions to each other, their personal and professional expectations, their communication process and any problems it may raise, the relevant dimensions of a contract to work together, their theoretical orientations and any differences between them, their views of the patient–therapist bonding process, and how stresses that arise will be handled.

In the real world, where staff and administrators are pressed for time and often have insufficient staff, the critical issues in the evolution of the co-therapy relationship may not be addressed in an ideal manner. An awareness of these limitations can facilitate the best use of the time and the resources available and lead to planning realistic treatment objectives for clients in group treatment.

There may be other critical relationship dimensions or co-leader–group management tasks that are not addressed in this theory. However, we believe that co-therapists must learn to perceive and appreciate the complexity of forces in the co-therapy relationship that affect the growth of their groups and their clients. Most importantly, we believe that groups should be co-led by therapists whose relationship has been developed to a collaborative level of functioning (Phase 3 and beyond). Such a team provides a rich, generative resource to the group as well as a model of a growing relationship. Even more importantly, such a team produces changes in clients that have far-reaching consequences for the rest of their lives.

# • 8 •

# *An Intimate Model for Co-Therapy* ★

## ROBERT L. GOULDING and
## MARY McCLURE GOULDING

BOB: Mary's very, very bright. Very perceptive. She has a lot of good things to say. She does a beautiful job obtaining the essential history in the early part of the work. I'm inclined now to sit back while Mary does the piecing out of the important issues. I think about what the script is—and what the payoffs are. Then I come in later. Mary does more of the early work. We've just been a good team. I wasn't looking for anybody when we got together.

MARY: I enjoy Bob's brightness—and his great lovingness, which he shows in his work. It is obvious to everyone that he cares what happens to the clients. Quite the opposite of the cold, analytic model. In all our writing, we've never written about co-therapy. We figured out the design for redecision therapy which is the therapy we practice. But we've never before analyzed the design of how we work together. We're very focused on what's going on for the patients and the group.

★Robert L. Golding, M.D., and Mary McClure Goulding, M.S.W., practice redecision therapy which combines Eric Berne's transactional analysis and Fritz Perls' gestalt therapy. We interviewed them at their home on Mt. Madonna, California in February 1985. Their candid remarks clearly demonstrate that they have established their style of working together and their identity as a co-therapy team. They lead us through their process of development as individuals, therapists, and co-therapists.

That's why I'm having difficulty looking at what goes on between us. In our work it's clear that we are both following the same steps. That may be one reason why what we do appears so integrated. We are both looking for the contract, looking for the example in the present, looking for the example in the past, going to the past to see if the person can feel, think, or do something different, and then returning to the present to see how it fits.

BOB: Very often, we both start to say the same words because we are both using the same system. But it is true that we also can pace well with persons from different systems, as Mary does with Michael Conant.*

## DEVELOPMENT AS PERSON AND THERAPIST

MARY: I didn't know how to socialize as a child. I was essentially lonely. My family background militates against co-therapy. I was the oldest and the bossy one. I was not cooperative with my sisters.

I read all the time. I loved books, and I love characterizations, and I loved knowing about people that way. To me, doing therapy is like reading the world's most exciting novel. How's it going to turn out?

When I graduated from college, I wanted a job in the diplomatic service. I applied to the college in Washington, DC that is the training ground for the consular service and was told that they wanted only men. This is the story of my life—I am the oldest of five girls. So, I married, had children, stayed home, and was depressed.

When my youngest was three-years-old, I decided I needed a career. I'd been a volunteer worker in congressional races, and I wanted to become a lawyer and to lobby for liberal causes or be a lawyer for the American Civil Liberties Union. I'd have liked to have been a member of Congress. However, it was the same story. Women were not wanted. When I applied at Boalt Hall at the University of California at Berkeley, I was told, "We don't accept applications from women with children." There were no other law schools within commuting distance at that time. I decided I was tired of bucking the male system, so I went to the psychology department and discovered I'd have to start over as a sophomore, because I lacked courses that had to be taken sequentially. I suggested that since they were interested in experiments, how about letting me take all the undergraduate psych courses at one time? The worst that could happen is that I'd flunk out. They

---

*See "Integration of Different Approaches," below.

didn't think that was an interesting experiment. I went to the School of Social Work, and they said, "Fine!" and gave me a scholarship besides.

At the University of California, I decided on a Corrections major. I wanted to work with women who were in prison and pregnant. I didn't do that because I became more and more interested in the clinical sequence of the curriculum. I do have a theory about the low recidivism rate among women prisoners. They become pregnant and stay home raising criminals. I see this as an area of tremendous import. Women prisoners are still reunited with their babies, and no one helps them recover from their prison experiences, and no one helps them mother well.

I was a pseudo-psychoanalytic social worker. I did no groups and certainly no co-therapy until I met Bob. I did run some other groups with a couple of other people while I was working with Bob, and I didn't like the experience. One was a fraudulent contract with a psychiatrist in the clinic. He said he wanted to learn transactional analysis. In actuality, he wished to deprecate it, and that became readily apparent. I quit leading that group because we just did not get along. It was rather silly because I knew I didn't like the man when I first said I'd do it. I believe liking is the most important, underlying element in the co-therapy relationship.

The other person was Janie Sivertsen, who died in 1969. We did all right together. But she didn't like me to be funny. She was very serious and a very good therapist. I had to muzzle myself while working with her. I said for ages that I'd never be a co-therapist with anyone but Bob.

BOB: By the time I finished college, I'd read everything Freud had written. I really enjoyed Freud. I enjoyed the clarity and the development of Freudian analytic theory. I was turned on by his brilliance.

My psychiatry residency at Perrypoint, Maryland Veterans' Administration Hospital started just before my 41st birthday, so I wasn't a kid any more. I did all kinds of things nobody else would do because I didn't care what anyone thought. I knew they weren't going to throw me out. I just wanted to experiment.

I've enjoyed in medicine and now in psychiatry the task of creating new methods that are more effective. One of the reasons I studied transactional analysis with Eric Berne was that I was so dissatisfied with the results of so-called classic psychotherapy.

Berne did not want to do co-therapy with anybody or let anybody do co-therapy with him. He was egocentric. He was also a marvelous teacher. He could listen to an audio tape and pick up very important things. He could listen better than any other teacher I ever had. I learned from him how to be more effective by listening—and confronting what I heard—and not just throwing it away.

I agreed to a two year contract as staff psychiatrist at the Veterans Administration Hospital in Roseburg, Oregon to pay back the salary I had earned as a resident. Every weekend I commuted to be with my family in Carmel, California. It was then that I began my training with Eric Berne on Saturdays. I also began leading groups with my patients on the veterans' ward and private groups in Carmel to obtain grist to apply the training I was receiving from Eric.

Then I started changing. I became quite active in groups and did them alone until 1964. Then in 1964, Dave Kupfer, who had entered transactional analysis just a little before I did, approached me and asked me if I'd be his co-therapist in some groups.

MARY: That was a very interesting team. I was one of their patients in a group of trainees who wanted to learn transactional analysis. Dave was intellectually brilliant, and Bob was brilliant and had real feelings. They made an interesting combination and, I think, a good one.

BOB: We were very good. We did much teaching across the country. In the early days, Dave and I were the primary teachers of transactional analysis. Eric Berne gave us teaching assignments that he didn't want. He told me, "When I lecture, I get people mad at me. When you lecture, you turn people on."

I then began to train in gestalt therapy with Fritz Perls and Jim Simkin and a number of other gestalt therapists. I began introducing gestalt in our groups, and Dave didn't like it. He kept stopping the process.

MARY: I remember that. If Dave was not the star, he would interrupt whatever Bob was doing. That was obvious to group members.

BOB: We finally became tired of each other and split in 1967. We were co-leading eleven groups each week in Carmel and Menlo Park when we split up. Most of them had been my groups originally. I took all the people who wanted to come with me, and David took those who wanted to follow him.

MARY: I joined them in 1966, just before the split-up. I chose to stay with Bob.

BOB: At that time I was very busy. I was working 60 to 70 hours per week. I was glad for the help.

MARY: I was pleased to join them. They were doing extraordinary therapy. It was exciting! The whole thrust of contracts, the practicality of the approach, the emphasis on "What are you going to do differently?" was such a departure from anything I'd learned previously. TA made wonderful sense and the whole gestalt movement was thrilling. I was learning from Bob how to combine the two.

BOB: I brought a lot of my general practice beliefs into my psychiatric practice. Being close with people and enjoying friendships was important to me. I never worried about the classic dictum not to be friends with patients. For example, I had a group of alcoholics for two years in an experimental program. We played poker, bowled, and golfed together.

I had a very different kind of relationship with my patients than most therapists do because I didn't give a damn about the old belief system. I thought I could take care of anything that arose out of friendships, and I did.

### Establishment of a Co-Therapy Team

MARY: In the summer of 1966 Bob and I began doing a little co-therapy. We started full time as co-therapists in late 1967. Our working together was gradual. First we covered for each other. He'd take my groups when I was gone, and I'd take his.

BOB: In 1970 we established our center here at Mt. Madonna in the Santa Cruz Mountains. Our work in those days was on-going training plus occasional marathons on weekends plus an occasional one week workshop plus two or three on-going groups.

MARY: We've been working together for twenty years. Whatever problems we had in the beginning, we've worked through a long time ago. We don't have any ego problem about who works with which patients or jealousy about what the other does. Competition between us does arise in that we each know what is best. . . . .so we may yell at each other once in a while.

BOB: But it doesn't get in the way.

MARY: We sort of take turns giving in. It's not a big deal because I know that in another five or ten minutes I can go the route I wanted to go if that is still pertinent.

BOB: We don't take any bad payoffs from whatever happens in a group.

MARY: Co-therapy works for Bob and me because we enjoy each other so much. We enjoy being married.

## WHY DO CO-THERAPY?

BOB: We have a lot of fun being creative. We have a lot of fun suddenly seeing what the scene is, what the script is, what the games are. I believe we are far more humorous as a team than we are as individuals.

MARY: We're a good audience for each other. We enjoy each other, and we play to each other. The major fun element in working as co-therapists is that we each have someone who appreciates our efforts besides our clients. This is a salient point for co-therapy. If a therapist is treating clients, such as delinquents, who don't appreciate the therapist and don't give positive strokes, that is, positive recognition, then having a co-therapist is especially desirable. The need for appreciation can be fulfilled by the co-therapy relationship. Plus, good co-therapy models stroking for your clients. A good co-therapist makes therapy life a lot easier.

One difference in our styles is I love creating scenes and developing a fully detailed picture of what's happening for the client. Bob will sometimes stop this process before there's a scene, and his way works, too.

BOB: From a theoretical standpoint, Mary places more emphasis on scene construction than I do. I like to work off the energy of the patient. For example, if a man switches from "I" to "you" in speaking of himself, he has changed from a Child ego state to a Parent ego state. He'll say, "I'm so tired. . . . you work hard and don't have any fun." I'll say "fight back" right then because that's the impasse between his tired Child and demanding Parent.

MARY: And I'll say, "Shut your eyes and repeat those statements and go back in time." And he finds the scene. Either way is OK. Bob does a canvas with minimal strokes, and I have a more detailed canvas.

BOB: That's right. You'll go for the history and detail and I stay more in the pure gestalt.

MARY: They are different approaches, and both are important. It's good to have both in the session. The client can experience a richness not possible with just one therapist.

## DISAGREEMENTS

BOB: If Mary's doing a scene like that, it's OK with me. I'll come in to help set up a dialogue. We know we come from different places with different ideas. But we have very few disagreements on how to proceed because we respect the other's judgment. Our clients have the option to choose the path they find most helpful in the group. For example, I confronted a person the other day on something I thought was significant, and Mary said, "I don't agree with that." I decided to stop because it would be hard for me to pursue a tack she disagreed with. I decided to wait till later and see what developed.

MARY: Usually our differences are stylistic, and that's not worth discussing in the group. But if it's an important difference in how we interpret content, then we must discuss it openly. And sometimes Bob might say, "The reason I'm doing this is . . . ." and go right on. This can help the client clarify what is happening as well.

BOB: As a general rule it's OK to disagree. But it is important to disagree without getting into uproar, without displaying affect in the disagreement. Again, it is important that self-esteem is neither lost nor impugned by the act of disagreeing. If we'd fight about it passionately, I believe that would be harmful and serve no purpose.

MARY: We don't fight about *how* to do therapy. Bob and I will sometimes disagree on what the problem is for a particular client and how best to treat. But we usually discuss that outside the group.

Occasionally we will fight about certain kinds of clients. For example, one of us may be exasperated by a client, and the other can present the opposing view. Or we'll fight about how a client may manipulate one of us to the detriment of the other and the group. It's the kind of fight that parents have about children when one person just can't stand one of the kids at that moment. But that kind of fight is rare.

BOB: Sometimes my family of origin gets in the way. My brother is three and one half years younger and fiercely competitive like me and a negative stroker. When Mary negatively strokes me, and she's usually not aware of doing it, I get angry and tell her about it.

## COMPARABLE AND COMPATIBLE

MARY: Our bias is that co-therapists must have *comparable* skills. However, they do not have to be the *same* skills. Both must feel equally OK in front of a group. Co-therapists need to applaud each other's contributions.

BOB: Co-therapy is possible if the co-therapists' belief systems are not incompatible. The belief system is the core of each clinician's work.

You must believe in your work in order to be any good as a therapist. It would be very hard for me to work with a psychoanalytic therapist who believes you must have transference from your patient in order to get the job done. I don't believe that. I believe transference gets in the way and takes too long to unravel. I just don't believe in augmenting and fostering transference.

MARY: I would encourage two people to combine their discrete skills if they do share a common belief system. Two conditions that allow this combination are: Both must be autonomous and both must have their own thoughts and feelings.

You must receive a gift from your co-therapist, or there is no point working together. If I am the only one giving, co-therapy simply will not work. Gifts must be traded all the time if the co-therapy relationship is going to work. The most important gift for me is an intellectual one. I want to learn from my co-therapist. The other gift is positive strokes of appreciation.

Be sure that you do not take away from your co-therapist. For example, I used to steal Bob's punch line. That's not fair especially when he has done all the groundwork up to that point. The client would think I was a genius, but it brought out hard feelings at break time. I learned to stop that by listening to the tape after the group sessions.★

Often co-therapists will be able to catch their mistakes on tape if they listen. That can be useful in addition to consulting with others, because you can hear yourself in a different way than you can while you are working.

BOB: If you want to change the subject during the group, say so and don't just do it. Let your co-therapist know by saying, "I want to take this somewhere else, is that OK?" Don't just take off into the heavens leaving your co-therapist behind.

Do not work your own problems out in the group. If you get angry over co-therapy in group, do not work it through there. Take it someplace else for supervision and help. They don't pay you to work out your problems in front of them. That's unethical behavior.

MARY: Speaking out directly to your co-therapist immediately after a group is important for the relationship. "You cut me off three times . . . !" We do that outside of group. But again, positive strokes

★This is consistent with our belief that co-therapists need to be more conscious of how they work together in the beginning. Later there is less need to observe the interaction between themselves: hence, there is more time for the clients.

must be there, or who would accept criticism and still enjoy co-therapy?

Bob: I don't think it's possible for people to be co-therapists if they don't like each other. I couldn't do it with anybody I didn't like. It's like an intense love affair, whether it is sexualized or not. Otherwise, there's not enough spark in it.

## CO-THERAPY IS NOT A TECHNIQUE

Bob: Co-therapy is not a technique but a way of operating as therapists. It is a relationship integral to the therapy process. If you define technique as a trick or artificial maneuver, then good and effective co-therapy can never be a technique.

Mary: If you mean by technique that a co-therapist will somehow behave differently than when he or she is the sole therapist of a group, then co-therapy is clearly not a technique. I am not appreciably different when working alone than when I work with Bob. We don't plan in advance the way we intend to be in a group, although some therapists we know practice this regularly. At most, I may say to Bob, "Make sure that on Sunday morning this person deals with this issue because I may let it slide." And sometimes one of us will say to the other, "I'm at an impasse with this person. Can you help?"

Bob: Co-therapy is a living process. It's an essential relationship. The number one reason I started doing co-therapy with Dave Kupfer was my loneliness. I was delighted to have someone to work with.

## EXPERIENCES WITH OTHERS AS CO-THERAPISTS

Mary: I don't do much co-therapy with others, because Bob and I are a team. Once a year, Muriel James and I run a one-week workshop together, which is lovely for us. We pick one of our favorite places, Akumal, Mexico, and we snorkel a lot between group sessions. We work effectively together and give each other plenty of space because our emphasis is different but complementary. She does more ego-state reconstruction, which is her self-reparenting therapy, and I do more redecision work. Both of us are at ease with each other's material. I have done women's groups with Joen Fagen, Irma Lee Shepherd, Barbara Hibner, Ruth McClendon, and Miriam Polster. I just finished a very interesting women's workshop with Michiko Fukazawa from

Tokyo. The participants were from Japan, Australia, Mexico, and the United States. With all of these people, I learn new methods and enjoy new experiences.

I also like working alone. I like running the show. There's something to be said for being able to set it up myself. But it's much harder work than sharing with a co-therapist, even one whom I am not that familiar with.

BOB: Fritz Perls and Jim Simkin were co-therapists at Esalen most of the time Fritz was there. Irma Shepherd and Fritz did workshops together. Joen Fagan worked as co-therapist with Fritz at Esalen. Fritz used a lot of co-therapists. When they were training people at Esalen, Jim Simkin and Fritz were both there when someone else was the therapist—and they would interrupt, come in, be obnoxious, or be helpful. That was like having three therapists at a time. At Esalen I didn't do much co-therapy with Fritz. I could get along with him all right.

I've done a couple of marathons, a three day and a five day, with Virginia Satir. I enjoyed working with her. The only problem I had co-leading with Virginia was she wanted to work all night. I'd get tired and quit.

The first long workshop we did here at Mt. Madonna was in June 1970. Virginia, Mary and I conducted a multiple family workshop. It was a three week experience, and Virginia stayed for two.

MARY: It was fun, exciting, and I thought we did well together. Virginia no longer works late into the night either. Age does take care of enthusiasm.


## MALE–FEMALE ROLE MODELS

MARY: I believe that my way of working with women co-leaders and men co-leaders has to do with my own growing–up experiences with siblings. I did not have to compete with my little sisters. I did compete with my male cousin and was very jealous of him because he was male. When I work with women I am nicer, sweeter, and certainly less raucous than I am when co-leading with a male. I am at my peak in skills only when I am doing a workshop with Bob. With Bob I can "let go" and feel as if I am flying, because I know that he is there and he will be the safety net if one is needed. I like women's workshops, because in them we combine teaching, exercises, and psychotherapy. I don't feel competitive, and I experience a tender mutuality as women join together to help each other grow.

When Bob and I work together, participants say that one of the best aspects of the workshop is our modeling of our relationship. We model caring and independence, but I don't think we do stereotypic role modeling, such as one being "hard" and one "soft."

BOB: I will be very hard and tough when people are doing things that are self-destructive like eating too much or doing things that will kill them or hurt someone else. In those kinds of confrontations, we take turns being the tough one. While Mary works, I'm following the process to know what's going on, as Mary does when I am working.

MARY: Certainly it's important for men to see males behave differently than they are expected to. Women will say to me, "You're such a good role model." It's interesting that men do not say that to Bob. My theory is that women know they're supposed to have role models, and men think they're supposed to do it on their own.

## INTEGRATION OF DIFFERENT APPROACHES

BOB: I could not work with anyone who says, "How does that make the group feel?"

MARY: You are able to work with Erv Polster, and he uses phrases like, "How does that make you feel?"

BOB: He is careful around me. And he has lots of other things to give.

MARY: I do believe you can integrate the work of therapists with discrete skills. For example, Michael Conant and I co-led a workshop once, and I thought we did a splendid job. It proved to be a very exciting and liberating experience for both of us. We have totally different skills and we overlap in the area of gestalt. His strength is bio-energetics, a body work therapy, and I don't do body work. I remind myself I should watch breathing and posture, but that's as far as I get.

We decided to alternate clients in the workshop so we could watch each other work. We didn't tell the group this beforehand. I discovered that while he was doing body work with clients, I could ask them certain things that proved helpful to them. And after Michael was through with a piece of work, I found I could make pertinent observations. We'd do fun things. For example, I'd say to Michael, "This person needs bodywork." Then Michael would say, "What's your thinking on that?" And I'd say, "Because I don't know what the hell to do with him."

## VIGNETTES OF OTHER CO-THERAPY TEAMS

MARY: The group knows everything. Of course, the group knows how people relate. The group knows if there is a real therapist and a pseudo-therapist. They can see that the trainee lacks the knowledge of the supervisor and the relationship is not equal. I'll give you an example. Many years ago we were in Argentina. A therapist had invited us down to watch his group. He had a male therapist trainee also in this group. The group was a homogeneous selection of beautiful, rich females. They each came in, one at a time, shook his hand and said, "Good afternoon, Doctor," but they all hugged the other therapist. And this difference was never addressed in group. Obviously, Dr. X was the brain, and the other therapist was the sexy one.

BOB: I did one marathon with my daughter once, but it was clear she was the assistant therapist, not the co-therapist, in our group. She simply didn't have my experience or the status in the group.

When a trainee is co-leading with a supervisor, he or she is an assistant therapist. It's not co-therapy to my mind. It is clear to everyone in the room that it is not co-therapy.

MARY: I agree. If you have an assistant therapist, I believe you must be honest and clearly label that person as such. I'm sure that AGPA members in your study who train students in group do just that.* I can see a problem if you pretend there is equality. We have a number of therapists who come to us because they want their spouses to be their co-therapists. The spouse has no training, but the co-therapy is intended to legitimize or enhance his or her standing. It's sometimes incredible to watch what happens when a couple pretends an equality that doesn't exist.

For example, one guy does a remarkable job of moving around his klutzy wife so that she actually looks good. But it's not co-therapy. Another example is the untrained wife who functioned so much more adeptly than her psychiatrist husband. This disparity was a contributing factor to their eventual divorce. The wife went on to get a PhD and became a therapist in her own right.

And then there was the therapist whose wife began working as his "co-therapist" when she was 65 years old. Her husband would suddenly say to her in group, "Honey, shouldn't the cat be out?" or "Honey, bring me a cup of coffee." Of course, he was 70 years old at the time, and this was their relationship. We had to be very careful

*Based on a 1983 survey of American Group Psychotherapy Association members. See Appendix.

selecting people we sent to him for training. Most women in our training program would be terribly upset by that kind of "co-therapy behavior."

## CLIENTS AS "CO-THERAPISTS"

BOB: Any good, active group therapist will encourage his or her patients to be observant, aware, and confrontive. In that sense they can become "co-therapists." For example, Erv Polster and I co-led a group at the AGPA conference one year for master group therapists. We had 32 people. If we had let them continue the way they began the process, it would have been a big fiasco. Each person's comment was different than the one before. They weren't listening to each other, and they weren't being congruent. We stopped them because it was a shambles. As co-therapists, it was our job to teach them how to interact appropriately.

MARY: When we do encourage clients to be our "co-therapists," we establish guidelines such as the following:(1) If you have a hunch, be direct and say it. Don't question people until they guess your hunch. (2) If you have a hunch, always give your evidence. (3) If the patient doesn't confirm your hunch, stop there. You may be projecting your own material, or the patient may not be ready for your hunch.

It's a magnificent idea to make one of your clients your "co-therapist" in the Youth Authority. The kids tend to do battle with their therapists. But if they know they will each have a time as "co-therapist," they'll all be more cooperative.

I think it's a good idea to teach your clients to be good therapists. It helps them cure themselves and let's them learn that not everyone reacts similarly to the same stress. They will start hearing themselves tell others to do the very things that they must accomplish.

## TRAINING THERAPISTS

BOB: At this time, we are doing almost all our work with therapists. This means we are dividing our time between therapy on one hand and supervision on the other. When we're doing therapy, we're almost always doing it together. If we're leading a big workshop, I might do more supervision, and Mary might do more individual therapy with the group. My primary goal is to train therapists. I love supervision.

MARY: And I love therapy. We don't do supervision as well together.

I believe it's too many voices for the trainee to absorb. And we do not always agree on how to supervise.

Bob and I designed our own way of teaching, which is peer supervision. All people who do training with us lead groups with each other. They each take turns being therapist.

BOB: I videotape for feedback to the trainee. We keep the period under review to twenty minutes and critique everything that went on during that time. In this way, we provide individual supervision of each therapist's work with the group.

MARY: I have half the group in the center with a designated therapist and group. The other half sit behind, and each has a separate assignment: look for ego states, games, stroking patterns, etc. After a 30 minute group, we spend about 45 minutes discussing it. Observers are to look for "What was done well?" and "What other options could be taken?" as well as their own assignments.

BOB: By living with our trainees for two or four weeks, we become privy to the games each plays. We get to things much faster than we could in individual therapy or once-a-week group therapy. We see what they do over and over again. We can get to the center of their pathology by watching how they operate. The trainees all know that whatever goes on during their stay here is appropriate to bring up in the context of their group sessions. There are no secrets.

MARY: Our therapy is based on the assumption that the patient is autonomous and will continue to be autonomous. We work with fairly high functioning individuals, and we presume they can give the protection and permission they need to themselves. They do not need us to function as parents.

We are primarily teaching people how to be therapists. They should already know diagnosis and be skillful in their own way of working with clients. We do not take responsibility for their clients as supervisors do. We see our trainees in workshops of a week or more or in ongoing training six weekends a year. That's time enough to teach them a few of our skills. But the decisions they make in their own offices about something like transference will depend on their style, their training, and the kind of clients they see.

BOB: I teach therapists how to avoid transference because that is not redecision work. For instance, every time a therapist says "tell me," he or she is asking for transference. And I teach them how to say "Will you do this?" without saying "tell me," "show me," or "do it for me." The use of the pronoun "me" gets in the way of the patient's treatment.

## TRANSFERENCE

BOB: When therapists train people to please therapists rather than please themselves, I believe transference is dangerous. The patients can be merely adapting to you as therapist rather than pleasing themselves. As therapists, we do not want a redecision from the Adapted Child in the person because that is not a change in behavior but a repetition of the old behavior.

We are not modeling being parents, but we are modeling closeness. We are not being close to each other just so people will say, "Wow, look how close they are!" We *are* close to each other, and that becomes a therapeutic tool. We don't design it that way; it's just part of the process.

MARY: People are in residence at our house while they do training with us. There's no question that it's a positive experience for them. They stroke each other and become very close. They have evenings to play together and talk, away from the everyday pressures of their lives. Many therapists have difficulty with closeness, and this is an opportunity to confront their difficulties directly and learn new ways of being close.

We see ourselves as facilitators, not parents. When the patient is transferring his or her parental images onto us, we do not encourage it or let it flower. We take the transference and return to the original source. We ask four questions: "What do you feel in one word?" "What do you say in your head about others in your life?" "What do you say in your head about you?" "How was it like that for you in your past?" And the person is right back to the source of the transference.

BOB: We do this because we believe we can accelerate the speed of the cure. It takes seven or eight years to break through a neurotic transference, and we can do it directly going to the source in seven or eight minutes. We believe in divesting the transference and going back to the original impasse, the actual scene where the person is stuck.

There is an important difference between transference and role modeling. When people respond to us with genuine affection and like us, that is not the same as responding to us as if we were their real parents. They are responding to us because we are warm, intimate, and loving, and we're doing it in the here and now. It's a mistake to consider that liking the therapist is always a manifestation of transference. I think transference often gets in the way of a cure. With positive transference, people will consume their time figuring out how to please you and not themselves. A negative transference slows the whole process down.

## MISTAKES

Bob: Most mistakes are not "mistake" mistakes in psychotherapy. If I make a mistake and I'm aware of what's going on, I can fix it. And I usually do. One of the things young therapists will do is harass themselves rather than acknowledge and fix the mistake. A skillful therapist will hear that what was said or not said was inappropriate and will do something to correct it. I tell trainees, "Don't worry so much about what you say—say it and see what happens."

## LISTENING

Mary: I am usually a creative listener. So, if I find myself not listening, or if I become bored as I listen, that is important information. First, I ask myself if it is my problem. I may be concerned, for example, with a personal problem. Then I ask myself if this person is boring or hard to follow. I might even say to the group, "I wasn't listening. Did anyone else have trouble listening?" I'd make that particular intervention very rarely, because I want the group to be an instrument of positive, not negative stroking.

Bob: When I'm working by myself, I very rarely wander off into my own mental processes. If I do wander off at these times, there is *always* a reason. So I might say to a person, "When you said such and such, suddenly I stopped listening to you. Does that happen very often to you, that people stop listening?" I bring it back to what was happening between us at that moment.

When I work with Mary, I do allow myself to wander off sometimes. That's both an advantage and a luxury of co-therapy.

## GROUP PROCESS

Bob: A lot of group process occurs in our groups in terms of how people interact with each other and how they may see others as sister or father. But we are not using that as our primary therapeutic model. We define what people do in a group as a part of their life script and the games they use to support that script.

We use group process, but we do not define it in the way that psychodynamic therapists do. Essentially, we do one-to-one therapy in the group. Most of the group process observations we make are based on our experience of people during their residence here, outside the group sessions proper.

MARY: We set the format for individual treatment in a group and teach our people how we want them to behave, as all therapists do. We function as the leaders, and after an individual piece of work is completed, the group functions as a means of positive reinforcement for the changes in the person's life. Also, group members will function as "co-therapists" when they observe and report things we miss.

BOB: The group is a tremendous support for people during a change process. When I first went into my own individual therapy, I had no idea what other patients in therapy were doing. I had no idea if people really made changes or not, and I had no way of judging its effectiveness. In group, everyone sees when people make changes.

## HAZARDS OF CO-THERAPY

MARY: The chief hazard for co-therapists is failure to be honest with each other. When that happens, a co-dependency develops within the co-therapy system as one person must deny his or her own experience of and feelings about the other. Pretty soon the denial system will take over so that the two of them cannot look honestly at what is going on. Trying to be nice is a big hazard, since it can induce co-dependency instead of co-therapy.

BOB: Another hazard is for co-therapists to play games with each other. There are many psychological games. The patients probably, without awareness, will feed into any game the co-therapists play. Then, they will attempt to solve the co-therapists' problems rather than their own. One of the biggest advantages of supervision is to help therapists work through their own games. This is especially true for co-therapists. A therapist must have identified his or her own games and have them under some control before becoming a co-therapist.

MARY: The people we train will often talk about their troubles with their co-therapists back home. The most common problem we hear is the passive–aggressive problem in which one therapist plays the game of "Nag Me" and the other tries to get the first to talk. One is silent, and one is active. If I'm the silent one, I resent the active one, because if he or she weren't so active I tell myself I would be. And if I'm the active one, I resent the silent one for "making" me be so active. Both feed into this process to create a stalemate. The game then becomes "If It Weren't for Her or Him." This is very difficult and not easy to resolve.

Usually we discuss how to have an amicable "divorce" as working partners.

The co-therapists who attend our workshops together are usually married. We're able to do more with these folks because they are both present. Their problems, of course, stem from early family experiences, and they can resolve their co-therapy issues by resolving their early pathological decisions. Otherwise, they can decide that they prefer to work alone. The bottom line is this: If you are not having fun with your co-therapist, for whatever reason, have a no-fault divorce. A lot of mental health clinics don't understand this principle. They assign people to do co-therapy, which is a misguided practice. It's hard for the patients when they experience a poisonous atmosphere. It injures the self-esteem of the therapists because they both will feel somewhat at fault, even if they do project the blame onto their co-therapist when the therapy goes awry.

Co-therapy is a little bit like co-parenting. If it's a rich relationship, it's good for everybody, parents and kids. But if it's not, then both parents and kids suffer. If the parents can't make it richer together, then it's probably best for each parent to take care of the children alternately, even though it's more work.

People whose major problem is differentiating self from other should begin treatment individually with one therapist. At first, it could be threatening for a patient to share a therapist. I believe that talking with two therapists can threaten his or her sense of self at that time. Later, when self boundaries are better defined, co-therapy can be applied.*

## ADVANTAGES OF CO-THERAPY

MARY: One of the disadvantages of a single therapist is that he or she will take one tack and may miss important things. A second therapist is apt to see things differently and offer a choice of interpretations.

Co-therapy is a learning device all through one's professional life. I would recommend a couple of groups and a couple of co-therapists for that reason alone. I learn from my co-therapists. Even today after twenty years of working with Bob, he still can teach me so much!

BOB: Co-therapy is more fun and less tiring, and that's most important for me. The excitement of two people enjoying work together is more important than whatever therapeutic effect it has.

*This is how we treated Christine in Chapter 6.

We teach and do therapy as our life occupation. Why should I risk burnout and loss of enthusiasm when it's so much more fun to do it with Mary?

MARY: This weekend I'll be doing a three day workshop in Salt Lake City. I will only do therapy and will explain the process after each piece of work. I know that (*sigh*) somewhere along the line I'll think, "God, I wish Bob were here."

Sometimes when it looks like every road is blocked, and Bob is there, I'll say, "I give up." Then Bob can take over and say, "I won't give up yet." Then the client begins to work effectively. Of course, no one wants *both* parents to give up.

BOB: And when I'm not involved in a particular power struggle, it's much more clear to me what's going on. That's a big advantage for both therapists and clients.

MARY: Patients can become "unstuck" with a new voice and a new approach. That's when I particularly long for a co-therapist. If I'm alone, I may say I don't know where to go, or I may play the tape back for review, or I may ask, "What do you feel; what do you say in your head about me; etc.?" But for me none of this is as good as having another person there to go on. The other time I most appreciate a co-therapist is in the afternoon when I'm growing tired. There's a time in the afternoon when I don't track. It's similar in my writing. There's a time when I must leave the typewriter. But if Bob's there, I don't get tired.

Our clients claim the major advantage for them in co-therapy is role modeling. They like to watch two people who have been together this long and who are able to argue and then laugh with each other ten minutes later. The mind set of many people is that if parents fight something terrible will happen. Their parents did not know how to resolve fights, and they don't either. They also get to see an intimate relationship.

BOB: We have more ideas to offer as a team than either of us does alone. We're two very intelligent people who know what we're doing and come at the task from different perspectives.

MARY: Intimacy in co-therapy is little things for us, like smiling or patting each other. We enjoy each other's brightness. I really like it when Bob does something different and outstanding.

BOB: Part of the process of therapy is teaching people how to be close with each other. That's always part of the therapeutic contract. Because we model closeness, we are able to help them achieve it.

MARY: My most awful day occurred when we had a workshop here at Mt. Madonna. My daughter was attempting a home delivery that didn't work. She'd gone to the hospital and I was really concerned. Was the baby going to die, or was she going to die? I co-led for a while, pushing it aside, and then I said, "I'm going to the hospital." And Bob just took over. That's an advantage of co-therapy. If I hadn't had a co-therapist, I would have had to stop the workshop.

BOB: One of my worst days was the day Fritz Perls died. Mary and I were doing a workshop at her place in Carmel Valley. I had dozens of friends who didn't know where I was or how to reach me. I learned about it through the newspaper. It was a terrible shock to me. We were very, very close. I kind of withdrew from the world. I was out of it that day. I was there, but I didn't function well, and Mary carried the ball. And then I suffered again when Jim Simkin died last summer. We were doing co-therapy that day, too. I just said to the group, "I'm mourning today and crying."

MARY: I have a more cheerful example. All my life I've wanted to travel. I finally got to do it in 1972 when we scheduled a world tour. We were leaving on that trip right after we finished a weekend training on Sunday. I was so excited that I simply couldn't hear anything they said that Sunday morning. Absolutely nothing they said was relevant. And I wasn't aware of it. Finally, Bob said, "Will you just stop working?"

BOB: That's a major advantage of co-therapy. If one therapist is out of sorts for some reason or just can't function that day, the other can do the job.


## WHO BENEFITS MOST—PATIENTS OR THERAPISTS?

BOB: As in any field, experience is a key. I would not expect anyone just starting out in co-therapy to be as effective as he or she might be in two or three years. Over time the positive advantages will start to be appreciated by your patients as long as both therapists avoid games.

MARY: I believe co-therapy adds richness and is a great benefit to patients. Our pacing and division of labor add richness, too. Neither of us has to be all things to all people.
There is someone else there. If I'm being confrontive, he can be supportive. If I'm being fast, he can slow down.

BOB: Co-therapy is not necessary to accomplish the work of therapy, but it's so much more fun.

MARY: A major thing we find is that people are afraid of any disagreement. With co-therapists they can see that disagreements do not end up in violence or divorce. This may very well contradict their family-of-origin experience. They also can break the belief that if only they'd been different, we wouldn't have disagreed. They learn that they did not cause our disagreement. We can help them understand that. We can resolve the transference on the spot.

BOB: Here's a classic example of how we operate as co-therapists. I was going to say something a few minutes ago. But Mary started speaking, so I stopped and waited. And now Mary is saying what I wanted to say.

# ◆ 9 ◆

# Therapists and Parents as Models for Being Human*

## VIRGINIA SATIR

In a family, two people come together and produce one person, a child. When those two are truly related in a co-equal way, they both acknowledge their responsibility to the development of this new life. This is similar to the responsibility shared by co-therapists in family or group therapy. They provide two sets of arms and legs, two sets of eyes and ears. They can become springboards for one another and bounce off one another in creative ways. It becomes easier for them to do what they need to do because they can see more and be doubly aware.

Co-therapy requires people who have learned to stand on their own feet. It takes people who do not have to depend on others for their power and their validation. There are not too many people around like that.

For the most part, therapists have not been trained to be whole people. Most therapeutic education does not teach too much about becoming a person. Therapists must know about that. Instead, they have been trained to perform techniques. They have not learned how to find out if their techniques work. That is, they have not learned how to experiment and test the results of their experiments. Therapists who assume they can apply the same technique in every case are mistaken.

*We recorded these statements by Virginia Satir during informal conversations with her in February 1985 and June 1986.

Technique is merely a form to be developed and used a moment in time to accomplish a purpose and then cast away or cast anew before being applied it to another unique person. We can teach technique until the cows come home and still not produce the kind of people needed as therapists. We must tune the instrument—ourselves as people—so that we may use the encounter of therapy to its potential.

I now regard all therapy as learning. We are always learning from models. Like good parenting, co-therapy is related to solid family-learning principles. How the co-therapists behave with one another, how they use each other, how they manage their differences—these are all models for health in relation to the individuals and families under treatment. Therefore, co-therapy is not a technique but a way of modeling being human.

Let us look at the balance of skills therapists must possess in terms of three dimensions. First is the skill of being congruent about oneself. That means I know what I know, and I know what I don't know. If you have some knowledge I don't, perhaps I can learn. A co-therapist being so clear can say, "I don't know this; do you know it?" This question exemplifies what every good therapist does in therapy with his or her patients. It also expresses what a good teacher can do when leading a family or group session with his or her student therapist. Although the student learning to be a therapist lacks knowledge, experience, and status in relation to his or her teacher, both student and teacher can be equal in the degree to which they practice congruence. In this way, a student can attain equality as a person with a teacher.

Second is the skill of helping others build their self-esteem. One example is the ability to mirror people so they can see something that they do not see about themselves. As your co-therapist, I might say, "I believe that our client could see something about himself, if he could just take an extra step and look at what he is doing. Do you have an idea about how you or I could do that?"

The third skill is literal knowledge and experience. For example, I may be quite knowledgeable about child abuse, so when words and descriptions of the blood and the gore come out, I do not flinch. I feel for my client and know that I have had some success with people suffering like that. But then you come in as my co-therapist, and you have never heard of such things. You may be sickened and do not see any hope whatsoever. You are not likely to be much help in the therapy at that point. However, you are being congruent with your lack of experience. Everybody has to start someplace. As a co-therapist, my role would be to help you to understand the client's predicament and share my belief that something can be done. I may have to do that for several sessions or perhaps just one session.

If we proceed with the idea that what we need in treatment are models for people, then the male–female model is a natural one for co-therapy. It models what you want to teach people. In practice it has not succeeded because a lot of co-therapy presents a dominant therapist and a submissive therapist. If, for example, the woman in the co-therapy team is relating toward the man as a placating person, the co-relationship will lose its value. I have seen nurses and doctors operate this way; I have seen husbands and wives attempt co-therapy; and I have seen social workers and psychiatrists team up. In these role designations there can be value judgments implied about who is better.

Historically, in the 1930s and 1940s, women were shown unequal treatment in their school and job opportunities. This was the experience of women who are now the leaders in the field of psychotherapy. It is important for women of the present generation to know that. The social context affects women and men as they work together. This is important because it touches the very essence of co-therapy. When women are treated as inferiors and buy it, they can never be good co-therapists. This is a feminist issue and also a clinical issue for co-therapy. It is easy to see how the co-relationship can be invalidated. It is desirable to give a model of how a male and a female can be together in a state of equality.

We must articulate the distinctions among role, gender, and value. As it stands, roles have a value in society. We must dissociate role from the notion of value and associate it with the notion of function. You do not get your value as a person from your role, and you do not get it from your gender. You obtain self-esteem from your own congruence. Gender is simply a given. Role is a function at a particular moment in time and not a description of a person. Value is related to a particular person and is a different thing entirely. This can be demonstrated by the healthy male-and-female co-therapy model. Each has a different gender, sometimes different roles, yet each is always of equal value.

Many therapists employ students and trainees as co-therapists, and this is shown by the 1983 survey of AGPA members. My belief is that the trainee is an apprentice in the presence of a therapist. In that case, I am the trained therapist and you come as an apprentice to be a part of the process. But very clearly, the apprentice is in a learning capacity. The therapist must define what that means and define it clearly to the group or family. You will construct a position of equality when everything is clear. The roles must be clear to all involved. If I am working with a male trainee, then he can be a marvelous student, and I can be the good teacher. That does not make me better than he is. We are equal in our sense of our value as persons. If he can feel good about being a student, he will have a great learning experience. I believe you can be a garbage man and yet stand equal to others in value as a person if you are clear about what you know and what you do not know, what you can do and what you cannot do, and you value yourself. It is an issue of how congruent you are within yourself and the degree of self-esteem you permit yourself. Clarity is the difference. Personal clarity allows equality to exist in the sense that a person is equal in value even though not equal in social status.

When I supervise people who are co-therapists with each other, I emphasize the necessity for equality in their relationship. Only when that is established can I then trust them with clients. In teaching the skills of co-therapy, I focus on the relationship between the co-therapists. Only when I believe their relationship with each other is congruent do I feel they can be effective and therapeutic and appropriate models.

I do not believe that co-therapy is the only way that clients can get something out of therapy. I do not think that co-therapy is the preferred way of working with families. Many therapists, including myself, do excellent work alone. Making hierarchical statements one way or the other is not helpful. I believe that families and groups can gain a great deal from having an individual therapist work with them. But that individual must have the ability to recreate the family. I use clients creatively to do that. It does happen that as I treat a family, one of its members becomes my "co-therapist." I can do that deliberately. As long as I make what I am doing clear, I can do many things of this nature. I will acknowledge their help and their co-assistance. The ones that I use most often are age four. They are the best. They will tell you what is happening.

Co-therapy teams do work well with one-parent families. They become a model for the family that was not there before. I have worked hard with such families, and I have often thought if there were a good male therapist to help it would be marvelous. One of the big problems we have in the world is how to bring up decent males. One of the things I try to do is to get males into men's groups and away from women. They have had enough of women in their upbringing. In men's groups, there can be male co-leaders and sometimes include a female co-leader.

## EVERY CHILD IS ASKED TO CHOOSE

In every family I have treated, the patient or child, whether grown up or not, was always between the two parents in some way. The child either was a link between them or divided them in some fashion.

Furthermore, each child was always asked on some level to make a choice between the two parents. That is true across all personality and diagnostic variables.* When this choice is free of rejecting components and indicates only a choice at a particular time, the relationship between parent and child can grow.

The child was connected to the woman's body, and it is so easy to think of the child as her possession. It is the woman who must give the man permission to be a parent. How does the woman give the male permission to parent? Obviously, she cannot do that unless she feels equal with the man and unless she believes he is someone who will treat the child well. The woman must believe she can connect with the man, that he has his feet on the ground. She must like who he is and know he has something to offer. She also knows she is not a man. Genders are different. Roles, as I have said before, are not the same as gender. A woman needs to be able to say to her baby, "You have a nice daddy!" Her arms must feel good and eager when she presents the child to his or her father. When the child is older, he or she sees the smile on her face when he or she is with Daddy. Then he or she also sees the smile on Daddy's face when he or she is with Mommy. By the time children are one year old they know all this.

I have done much therapy, as you can imagine. I have done co-therapy, and some of it has been just great. It was not great when there was an unacknowledged situation in which my co-therapist was trying to outdo me or challenge me or perform some other sabotaging maneuver. This is unhelpful competition. The same dynamic can disrupt parents' effectiveness. In these cases, the way I confront my co-therapist becomes a model for how our clients could do it in their own lives. I do all such confrontations in front of the family. That is the meaning of modeling. This does not repeat the action of parents who go into the bedroom to discuss what they are going to do about their child. It is the modeling that makes the most effective impact. On that level, I believe co-therapy adds a great deal.

## BENEFITS

Does co-therapy benefit the therapists more than the clients, or do the clients benefit more? That is a question that can never be answered. In some situations the therapists may gain the most. For example, co-therapy can be a support to a therapist and stem his or her loneliness.

---

*This is a salient point for co-therapy. Co-therapists must be aware that their patients will also choose between them.

There is a lot of loneliness among therapists. I imagine there is less temptation for a therapist to suicide if he or she is working as a team. But let us put it on a scale. If the therapists are gaining something, then chances are the patients are too. If you as a therapist do not think of what you are getting out of the therapeutic contract, then you are headed for trouble. Everybody must get something, and I believe that is possible. A healthy relationship between co-therapists benefits both therapists and clients. It makes the lives of co-therapists easier if they enjoy a good relationship. When there are two therapists, labor can be divided. It is similar to what happens in a healthy family. Mother has been home with the kids all day and says to Father when he comes in, "I just want to stretch out now, so you take over." It benefits the kids because they are not stuck with an exhausted parent.

I prefer to work with a male co-leader. I have worked with the same sex as well. Same-sex co-therapists encounter the same difficulties as Mother and the oldest daughter when they try to handle the whole family. One-parent families are replete with these issues, too. Same-sex co-therapists cannot mirror or model the same kind of wholeness that a male-female relationship can. However, they can offer arms and legs, and they can be congruent with each other. They can model how they deal with disputes and how they relate to each other's creativity.

When a husband-and-wife team conducts therapy, many of their own problems surface. The fate of the therapy depends on their own ability to confront this as it happens. It is that simple. I know that many people who are capable of confronting such problems directly give an authentic model for their clients.

I believe the most important thing in therapy is for therapists to understand themselves clearly and for them to see themselves realistically, so they will not project onto their clients. Showing the couple or family how you manage your own problems is one thing. However, there is also a point at which you may take advantage of a couple or a family and make them your therapists. When that happens, patients have to let go of what they want.

I'll give you an example. A man and woman who lived together were co-leading a family therapy session. At a certain point, the woman began to develop a lot of resentment toward her co-therapist. It was not in the woman's awareness that her resentment was directed toward her partner. Rather, it took the form of questioning his competence. She began attacking him during the session. She believed this was what she needed to do as a model. I interrupted that particular session because I knew it was not productive. I asked her what was bothering her. She said she was feeling that her co-therapist did not know what he was doing. I asked the family if they knew anything about this kind of experience, and, of course, they did. And I said, "Let's see what we can learn from it." Then I asked the male co-therapist how he felt about being seen as incompetent in relation to his co-therapist. He replied that he did not like it. Then he shook his finger at her and said, "You know, you do this to me all the time." At this point, I said to the therapists, "I don't believe we should take the time of this family in this way. It's clear that it belongs to you." These are always matters of clinical judgment. In this case, it helped to have an objective person to call the process for the co-therapy team.

An effective co-therapy team can provide objectivity for each other. For example, let us think about a stream—a stream in which people are boating. When they all feel that they are with the current they can sing and enjoy themselves. Suddenly, the boatman may decide to leave the flow of the current and turn against it. The passengers will experience the resistance against the flow. If the passengers are responsible and aware people, they will say, "Hey, we feel we are off course." They would do it lovingly. That might be enough to bring the boatman back. He might say, "Yes, I was taking a short cut."

We can adapt that imaginary scene to co-therapy. When a person is inside of something, he or she may not be as aware of the flow going on as a person looking on. A co-therapist can be that person looking on. I can imagine a male co-therapist becoming engaged in a fight with a male member of a family. Some of these fights lead someplace and some lead nowhere at all. His co-therapist can say, "Wait a minute, I don't think this is going anywhere. So let's stop and see what we are doing." Now if you must always take your co-therapist's side and believe he or she is always marvelous and does everything right, you must deny your gut feelings and shut up. But a person cannot really hide all that. Someone in the family will pick it up. They know when the boat is out of the flow.

## DIFFICULTIES

Co-therapy becomes more expensive because two therapists cost more than one. It also means people must be finely tuned with each other, and that requires an investment of time and energy by both therapists.

My first co-therapy experience was with a psychiatrist, and I knew more than he did. It was not a good experience. I was busy trying to do what I call man-save. I was not that sophisticated and knowledgeable about what my own family was like at that time, so I did not know I was a man-saver. He did not know anything as far as the family was concerned. But I wanted him to succeed and not to have hurt feelings. It was a mess. At one point, one of the patients said to us, "*You* ought to have therapy." And she was right.

I would have never believed the following experience could happen to me. Years ago, I agreed to co-lead a seminar with a man in Mexico whom I did not know well. As we were sitting at the swimming pool just prior to the beginning of the seminar, he said to me, "I consider women inferior." I said, "Oh?" and we went inside. This took me quite by surprise. You could not pay me enough money to do that seminar again. It was crazy. One particular woman, whom my co-therapist had really pushed, physically attacked him when the seminar was over. That was an example of negative co-therapy at work. It was like the house was flooding. I was going around seeing that the water did not drown everyone.

I shall give you another example of a hazard of co-therapy from my own experience. An analyst from New York asked me to come in and be his co-therapist to help him with a very difficult family. I knew it was a difficult family because I had watched him and the family on videotape. When I came in, no matter what I said or did, he just turned me off. I would make a comment, and, without acknowledging it in any way, he would immediately ask me to look at something else. He gave no recognition of my effort. After a while, I saw the family becoming "antsy." And pretty soon the family was in terrible chaos. I was furious with this man. I did not know what to do with him. Today, I would have acted differently. Here we were two therapists producing symptoms in the family. I told him afterwards, "As I think about it now, I would have liked to have hit you in the head for playing your arrogant role." What can you learn from such an experience? You can learn that the hazards come in any kind of co-therapy when the roles are not clear and when people are not living up to their agreements. In this example, we had fully discussed our agreements and my role. He wanted something from me, but he gave me no opportunity to give it to him.

Mistakes in therapy are usually errors born of arrogance. If you are arrogant, you will not look beyond yourself to see what you need. Some persons make definitive statements simply because they think they ought to. Some bad errors in diagnosis have been made this way. I think that when therapists believe they must act as though they know something when they do not, they are repeating old family myths and impeding therapy. A mistake is something one learns about after it has been done. One cannot know about a mistake ahead of time. However, I do know that if I show off, that is always a mistake. The only time I

ever was hit by a patient was in my early days, when I was showing off
to a group how deft I was in my communication with him. I was not
really trying to make a connection with him, and he resented it.

## CO-THERAPY IS A MEANS OF STARTING THE HEALING
PROCESS WITH TWO PEOPLE

Before I came west to California, in 1957, I read a paper by Don
Jackson, aiming toward a theory of schizophrenia (1957a). You cannot
imagine what the climate was like at that time. The whole world was
psychoanalytic. Then these freaks appeared, people like Murray Bowen, Nathan Ackerman, to name a few, and myself. Don Jackson was
part of an ethnology group at the Menlo Park Veterans Administration
Hospital, which included Gregory Bateson, John Weakland, Jay Haley, and Bill Frey. They were studying one family. Gregory Bateson
was interested in how information would come across to make people
crazy—the anthropology of it.

I remember fondly my association with Gregory. He was one of my
special people. I loved him very much, and I think he returned that to
me. Gregory understood life. He did not have much patience for
one-upmanship games. I think he understood what the double bind
was all about before anyone else because of his ability to watch what
was going on—to observe process. He also knew how to break the
double bind:(1) to comment on the discrepancy and (2) allow the
person to openly make the choice to be congruent. Gregory was one of
the true geniuses of our world, who understood first that life is sacred
and second that life is. He believed the way we live our life is always
something superimposed on life itself. He believed that life was always
manifesting itself and, further, that life always had a reason for manifesting itself. He watched life without judging. Gregory would begin
the inquiry into co-therapy this way: How do we start the healing
process? Do we start with one person, two people, or three? Co-
therapy is a means of starting the healing process with two people,
preferably a man and a woman, who have got their act together.

Three months after I arrived in California, I called Don Jackson, and
he invited me to come to a meeting of the group. That was February
1958. I brought with me seven years of experience with families I had
treated in state hospitals in Illinois. Don asked me if I would help him
form an institute. This was the beginning of the Mental Research
Institute (MRI). We joined our efforts for the purpose of studying
family interactions to discover what kinds of interactions promote
health and what kinds do not. By September we had a grant to train

people. Because I didn't really like the research, I developed the stances, those distinctive patterns of communication (placating, distracting, computing, and blaming) in a very short time to help my trainees learn to understand the process of families. There is a place for translating your experience into conceptual frames. But there is a great danger in never having the experience to test the conceptual frames you create. MRI was an opportunity to combine the two.

The training program offered an opportunity to explore co-therapy. At MRI, all my trainees were in male-female teams or units. I have felt from the beginning that the yin–yang or female–male of the person and of relationships had to be addressed. Each unit had its own families to treat. They were all capable of doing co-therapy. In addition, each therapist was able and willing to be an observer while his or her partner was handling the session. In the use of co-therapists I stuck closely to the model of the family, where sometimes one parent alone is carrying the parental load, sometimes two parents share it, and sometimes one parent says, "I'll watch and you take the responsibility."

Sometimes I would go in with one of the trainees and take on a co-therapy role. Then, on other occasions, they would enter as co-partners, and I would watch what they did. Whenever one attempts to change something, one benefits from having someone observe from the outside.

## ANY FORM OF THERAPY CAN WORK

Freud was always working in a triad within the individual, but he did not recognize it. Mother, father, and child are the primary triad. That is how the concept of transference and countertransference came to be. The therapist brings her or his triad into the treatment context, and that is part of the healing process. Somehow the therapist's mother and father are always involved in the process as the treatment proceeds.

I teach therapy in triads now. I do not work with dyads anymore. All my training is in triads. I believe the triad is the *complete human unit*. Three trainees make up each triad. All content and theory about how to work with human beings derive from the dynamics of the primary triad. If there are just two trainees, we still must return to the primary triad. The triad contains all the information about how the unit becomes a person. It contains information about how behavior is solidified in the individual and how trust is developed. These are triadic issues.

Every dyad, if it is going to live constructively, is a triad. In the linear or hierarchical model the pair becomes one—you or me—and the struggle is who will be superior. In the organic or nourishing model, the pair becomes three—you, me and us—and there is room for each one. The "us" is the relationship and is like a reflection of a primary triad: mother, father, and child. For example, your knowledge of your father is based on (1) what your mother told you about him, (2) how he treated you directly, and (3) how you saw him relate with your mother. And your knowledge about you mother is based on (1) what your father told you about her, (2) how she treated you directly, and (3) how you saw her relate to your father. How you saw your parents relate may be very different from what they told you. Every child understands such discrepancy. Furthermore, we must identify both with the sex we are and the interrelationship of the two sexes we came from. The "us" of a relationship is made up of how two people put their family triads together. That "us" is the context the next generation of children are born into. What we have in a relationship is the playing out of the two primary triads. There is always a fit somehow. So putting three therapists in training together stimulates the comprehensive understanding and working out of their primary triads. I do all my training in triads for this reason.

As a therapist, I am an initiator to help things manifest themselves. Let us suppose that whatever is there in a family is sleeping or hidden, and my job is to wake people up and expose what is concealed. I actively initiate this process so people do not go on struggling as they have before. There are blind spots in everyone. Not one of us can see ourselves as other people see us. One of the things therapists have in their favor is they can see what their clients cannot see. That is not because therapists are smarter; it is because they are in a different place. We must remember this in order to be humble and not arrogant. The same phenomenon is true for co-therapists. They can point out each other's blind spots.

In choosing a co-therapist, I look first for congruence. When I select people for my training group, I ask three questions and these questions have relevance for selecting a co-therapist.

1. Why do you want to join this program? That is my test for authenticity and directness.
2. As you look at yourself now, what do you see that still needs to be changed? That is my test for reality.
3. And then, I would ask myself: "Are they wearing their sexuality openly, vitally, and appropriately?" This is the test for looking at the wholeness of a person.

These three questions determine if the person is clear about his or her own reality, congruence, and sexual energy. Sexual energy is something that makes us feel alive. It does not mean we go to bed with everybody. Now if you add skill and experience, you have a winning combination.

We must remember that clients always present a system that is rooted in the status quo. There is always resistance to change because we must go through the known and into the unknown. That's why trust is so important. First, co-therapists need to be well grounded in themselves and each other to withstand the pressures of resistance, even though clients are "willing" to change. Second, there will be a period of chaos and disorganization that opens up the possibility for change. People do not know where they are going, so therapists must bear responsibility for what they as therapists are doing and where they are going. This is a paramount ethical issue for therapists because they have much power to influence and persuade at this point.

We must remember that any mode of therapy can work whether individual, pair, family, or group. Any form of therapy can work whether conducted by one therapist, co-therapists, or a triad. What is vital to me is the quality of the relationships that surround the form of therapy used. I would like people to know they are sacred and that they can act in ways that fit their sacredness. Self-worth is the only treasure we have.

◆ ◆

# *Appendix*

SURVEY OF THE AMERICAN GROUP PSYCHOTHERAPY
ASSOCIATION

*SURVEY OF THE AMERICAN GROUP PSYCHOTHERAPY
ASSOCIATION*

In 1983, we undertook a survey of the membership of the American
Group Psychotherapy Association in order to establish a data base for
current attitudes and beliefs among practitioners of co-therapy.* We
drew a random sample of 200 members and sent them a 15 point
questionnaire. Ninety-four persons responded, often with thoughtful
additional comments, which added greatly to the information we
received. We are grateful to our respondents for providing such rich
data on which to base our conclusions.

The content of the questionnaire was based on our readings in the
literature of co-therapy and augmented by the issues that grew out of
our own clinical practice with more than 50 co-therapists and trainees
in over 15 years. As expected, our survey generated new questions
which subsequent researchers can explore. The questionnaire in full
follows.

*We wish to recognize the generous support of the Mental Health Service of
Group Health Cooperative of Puget Sound, which made it possible for us to
conduct our research.

## CO-THERAPY QUESTIONNAIRE

1. For how many years have you practiced as a therapist?
\_\_\_\_ 1–2 \_\_\_\_ 3–4 \_\_\_\_ 5–6 \_\_\_\_ 7–10 \_\_\_\_ 11–15 \_\_\_\_ over 15
2. Are you: \_\_\_\_ Male \_\_\_\_ Female
3. What is your preferred mode of practice? (Please check one only.)

\_\_\_\_ Individual therapy          \_\_\_\_ Family therapy

\_\_\_\_ Couple therapy            \_\_\_\_ Group therapy

Other (Please explain) _____

_____

4. Is your practice primarily in (Please check one only.)
\_\_\_\_ A private practice
\_\_\_\_ A group practice with other therapists
\_\_\_\_ An agency or institution
\_\_\_\_ Hospital or medical center
5. What is your interest or experience in co-therapy?

\_\_\_\_ Have practiced co-therapy—for how many years? \_\_\_\_

Number of co-therapists worked with \_\_\_\_

\_\_\_\_ Have not engaged in co-therapy but plan to practice it in the future.

\_\_\_\_ Not interested in practicing co-therapy.

Why not? _____

_____

(Please skip to Question 13.)
6. If you have worked as a co-therapist, did you and your partner(s) choose to work together, or were you assigned to work as a co-therapist with another?
\_\_\_\_ I chose my partner(s)      \_\_\_\_ My co-therapist was assigned
7. What qualities do you (would you) look for in a co-therapist?

_____

_____

8. As a co-therapist, what assets do you (would you) bring to the working relationship? _____

_____

9. Have you worked with a co-therapist of the opposite sex?
\_\_\_\_ Yes \_\_\_\_ No
10. a. Do you prefer your co-therapist to be
\_\_\_\_ Same sex \_\_\_\_ Opposite sex \_\_\_\_ Equal preference

b. Why? _____
11. Will you (would you) do co-therapy with a person who is in training with you or under your professional supervision?
\_\_\_\_ Yes \_\_\_\_ No

12. In which modes of therapy do you (would you) practice co-therapy?

    \_\_\_\_ Individual therapy          \_\_\_\_ Family therapy

    \_\_\_\_ Couple therapy            \_\_\_\_ Group therapy

    \_\_\_\_ Other (Please explain.) _____

13. What are the most important factors in the success of a co-therapy team? (Please rank from 1 for most important to 7 for least important.)

    \_\_\_\_ Compatibility of the therapists' theoretical viewpoints

    \_\_\_\_ Equality of participation

    \_\_\_\_ Similar levels of activity

    \_\_\_\_ Complementarity of balance of therapist skills

    \_\_\_\_ Similarity in age

    \_\_\_\_ Similar levels of experience as therapists

    \_\_\_\_ Other _____

14. What are the principal hazards of co-therapy?

15. What are the principal benefits of co-therapy?

THANK YOU VERY MUCH FOR PARTICIPATING

## Results of the Survey

We were delighted to find that our sample was highly experienced. None of our subjects had less than 5 years of experience as a psychotherapist. Indeed, 72% had over 15 years experience in the field and 21% reported that they had between 11 and 15 years of clinical experience. Fifty-six respondents were males, 36 were females, and 2 were unidentified. Surprisingly, just 21 subjects stated that group treatment was their preferred mode of clinical practice, whereas 40 subjects indicated individual treatment as their preference. Fourteen subjects reported more than one preference. The majority of our respondents were in private practice, 62%, and the remainder practiced in hospitals, agencies, or other settings.

The responses to question 5 (interest and experience in co-therapy) showed this to be not only a mature sample but a highly sophisticated one in terms of experience with 'co-therapists. Eighty subjects stated that they had practiced co-therapy and 71 of them specified the number of years they practiced. Twenty-nine subjects had practiced 15 years or more as co-therapists. Of those specifying years, only 9 persons had practiced less than 5 years of co-therapy.

Those responding affirmatively favored a variety of co-therapy partners. Sixty-four of them specified the number of co-therapists they had worked with during their careers. Twenty-four persons had worked with between one and four co-therapists; 24 persons had worked with between 5 and 10 co-therapists; seven persons had co-led with between 12 and 16 co-therapists; six persons had collaborated with 20 co-therapists; and three persons had been with between 30 and 100 co-therapists.

One person stated he had never practiced co-therapy but "I find the concept interesting."

One person stated that he had practiced co-therapy for 7 years but "currently I am a Jungian analyst and I work in that mode most of the time."

Seventy-six therapists not only were experienced as co-therapists but also wanted to continue co-therapy practice.

Sixteen subjects expressed their disinterest in co-therapy. Of that group, 13 had never tried the practice, and three had tried but still were not interested. Their comments by way of explanation are of particular importance and are quoted below.

Those who have practiced but are not interested stated:

1. "Neither therapeutically advantageous nor cost effective."
2. "At present I prefer doing group alone."
3. "I would only use a co-therapist on certain occasions, special circumstances, or particular groups."

Those who have never practiced and are not interested stated:

1. "I'm too narcissistic. I don't share well."
2. "It's less hassle to practice solo."
3. "I am winding down my practice due to advanced years."
4. "It's too expensive for my clients."
5. "It's more expensive than rewarding to my patients."
6. "No suitable co-therapist available."
7. "I'm satisfied both personally and professionally to go it alone—except in the treatment of certain adolescents, where separate therapists are essential for both child and parents."
8. "It is cumbersome with time-scheduling problems."
9. "I have a real question as to its value and my suitability."
10. "It's too difficult."
11. "It's too complicated for the context of my practice."
12. "It's ineffective and inefficient."
13. "It's not indicated by my clientele."

From responses to question 6 we learned the following: 58 subjects always chose their co-therapists; 6 subjects always were assigned their co-therapists; and 17 subjects had experienced both choice and assignment. Thus, the experience of choosing a co-therapist was much more common than being assigned. This factor distinguishes our study from most previous research in the field, which relied on subjects who were assigned their co-therapists. Since nearly two-thirds of our sample were in private practice, it is not surprising that they were more likely to choose with whom they work than those in an institutional setting.

In response to question 7 (the qualities therapists look for in a co-therapist) we summarize the most frequent replies below.

| Number of responses | Quality |
|---|---|
| 22 | Equal in communicating and openness |
| 20 | Compatible, equal power, noncompetitive |
| 17 | Skills |
| 15 | Similar theoretical orientation/values |
| 13 | Sensitivity, empathy |

Seventy-eight subjects responded to this question. The data include more than one response for several subjects. It is informative to compare these responses with question 13 regarding the ranking of the most important factors in the success of a co-therapy team. The top categories in each summary of responses correlate positively.

In response to question 8 (the assets therapists bring to the working relationship) we summarize the most frequent replies below.

| Number of responses | Asset |
|---|---|
| 26 | Experience |
| 12 | Skills |
| 11 | Knowledge |
| 10 | Cooperation |
| 10 | Open communication with co-therapist |
| 9 | Flexible, willing to learn new approaches |
| 8 | Comfortable with self, based on competence and confidence |
| 7 | Sensitivity |
| 6 | Willingness to share and learn |

Seventy-four subjects responded to this question. The data include more than one response for several subjects.

In response to question 9, 80 persons stated they had worked with a co-therapist of the opposite sex, and only one had never done so.

In response to question 10a, the majority of our therapists preferred the opposite sex in their co-therapist choices, and this is shown in the summary below.

The number preferring opposite sex: 26 men and 21 women
The number preferring same sex: 1 man and 1 woman
The number expressing equal
   preference between the sexes: 20 men and 9 women

              TOTAL  47 men and 31 women

Among 31 women, opposite-sex co-therapy teams were preferred two to one; however, this was not a significant difference statistically (Chi square $= 2.4; P > .05$: Roscoe, 1969). We were unable to use the Chi square test of statistical significance for same versus opposite sex preference because the samples were too small (observed frequencies less than 5). Although the responses of "same-sex" were not statistically significant, they did represent idiosyncratic responses for our sample.

In response to question 10b, the most frequent statements are summarized below.

| Number of responses | Why they chose opposite-sex partners |
|---|---|
| 19 | Balance |
| 11 | Transference |
| 9 | Modeling |
| 7 | Parenting |

The data include more than one response for some subjects.

In response to why they expressed equal preference between the sexes, most subjects said "It did not make a difference" and did not elaborate further. One subject spoke for the majority: "I find sex of the co-therapist insignificant. The capacity to relate well is what counts."

In response to question 11, 70 of 80 subjects responding stated they would do co-therapy with a person who was in training with them or under supervision.

| | | | |
|---|---|---|---|
| yes | 70 | maybe, if ... | 3 |
| no | 7 | no response | 14 |

Psychotherapists in our sample approved 10 to 1 the use of students and supervised persons as helpers in the treatment dyad, although strong opposition was expressed by the seven dissenting votes. One of the seven objectors said, "This is not co-therapy; they are not equal in knowledge or experience. It works better for me to observe a person or to employ the videotape recorder."

Under the "maybe" category, one therapist reported, "Yes, but only as an *assistant* therapist," where it is clear that the relationship is not equal. Another said, "I have not done it, but I have shared a case with students that worked well." Presumably, this patient was treated both by the supervisor and the student in alternating though not conjoint sessions. Another "maybe" made an important distinction for therapists to consider, saying "yes to a trainee, but no to a staff person under my supervision." The questions appear to be "How equal do I want this person to become?" and "What risks am I willing to take?" For example, if irresolvable conflicts emerge, a therapist can send a trainee away, but he or she must continue to work with another staff member.

The willingness of our sample to employ students as co-therapists may be a function of our sample's characteristics, that is, a mature group of psychotherapists, many of whom may be said to be in the generative stage of their professional life. However, many articles in our bibliography testify to the widespread popularity of forming treatment dyads for the purpose of training.

In response to question 12, our sample showed a clear preference for group therapy as the setting for co-therapy, with 84% of our sample or 79 therapists responding affirmatively. Family therapy and couple therapy were the next choices, with 55% and 54% of our sample responding affirmatively. Not surprisingly, individual treatment was named by only 11 therapists. It is significant to note that co-therapy is practiced in individual treatment, and perhaps more frequently than previously recognized; recent publications corroborate a trend in this direction (see References). Sometimes it is quite helpful and informative to request a second therapist to be present for an individual hour with a client, especially during an impasse in the therapy, as one therapist specifically mentioned in our survey. Thirteen persons did not respond, and nine therapists attested to other modes and settings in which co-therapy proved helpful. Some of the appropriate treatments suggested were behavioral modification programs, combined individual and group with co-therapy, multiple family therapy and sexual counseling.

Question 13 asked respondents to rank-order the most important factors in the success of the co-therapy team. The rank order was determined by calculating the median scores for the various factors. These median ratings are given below in the left-hand column, with the number of therapists giving first-place votes for each in parentheses. Eighty-nine subjects responded, among whom eight marked factors but did not rank.

| Median rating | Factor | First place votes |
|---|---|---|
| 1.82 | Complementarity of balance of therapist skills | (32) |
| 2.13 | Compatibility of therapists' theoretical viewpoints | (23) |
| 3.14 | Equality of participation | (8) |
| 3.47 | Similar levels of experience as therapists | (2) |
| 3.73 | Similar levels of activity | (0) |
| 5.87 | Similarity in age | (0) |
| ---- | Other | (12) |

Twelve therapists marked "other" with first-place votes. Their remarks—several subjects made multiple comments—are excerpted and recorded as follows:

Compatibility of personalities and liking each other (mentioned three times)
Mutual respect (mentioned twice)
Rapport and mutual trust (mentioned twice)
Willingness to communicate openly to each other (mentioned twice)
Openness to process the co-therapy relationship (mentioned twice)
Compatibility of therapists as people
Professional maturity
Personal analysis
Can communicate honestly
Personal clarity

Another 18 subjects made comments under the "other" category to define their own criteria for success. Some are listed below:

"Intangible assets"
"That indescribable something—vitality"
"Liking each other"
"Ability to dialogue with each other"
"Willingness to be open with each other and patients"
"Comfortable with activity and passivity, dominance and subordination"
"Supervision or time to discuss co-therapy"
"Ability to work as a team"
"Compatibility of therapists' values and life orientation"
"In sophisticated groups, it's difficult but sometimes valuable to have varying theoretical viewpoints."
"Flexible give and take between therapists"

We analyzed all "other" categories and collapsed the majority of them into four categories; their frequency of expression is given in parentheses (several subjects made more than one comment each):

1. Openness in communication (9 comments)
2. Liking each other as people (5 comments)
3. Respect (4 comments)
4. Trust (2 comments)

These four categories are well represented in the 12 persons who cast first-place votes for "other." Based on this information, we supplanted three factors in question 13: similar levels of experience as therapists, similar levels of activity, and similarity in age. We replaced them with openness in communication, liking each other as people, and respect. In retrospect, had they been added to the original six factors given in our questionnaire, we might reasonably have expected a different pattern of ranking than we obtained. These criteria should be considered in future surveys of co-therapist behavior and attitudes.

In our interpretation of responses to question 14, we assumed that the principal hazards of co-therapy were related directly to the problems clinicians experienced during its practice. We report in detail on each of these hazards in Chapter 5. Ten major hazards were named by our respondents, and they are listed below along with the number of therapists who specified each.

| Hazard | Frequency of response |
|---|---|
| Competition | 28 |
| Countertransference | 16 |
| Differences | 11 |
| Dependence on co-therapist | 7 |
| Lack of communication | 7 |
| Transference | 6 |
| Not liking each other | 5 |
| Too costly in money | 5 |
| Unresolved conflicts | 4 |
| Too costly in time | 2 |

Other hazards reported included "performance anxiety" and "the painful exposure of one's limitations as a therapist to a colleague." Both comments indicate a reluctance to show less than outstanding ability, much less mistakes, to other therapists. Ironically, this tendency may increase with the skill and level and years of experience of the clinician, especially if the individual's "Be perfect" driving ambition is stimulated. There probably are people who refrain from co-therapy for these reasons. And yet, the professionals making these remarks have in fact practiced co-therapy and somehow pushed past their fear.

Five additional cautionary remarks were cited by our respondents:

1. "In couple therapy, co-therapists must be sure not to gang up against one person."
2. "Do not overwhelm clients by giving too much information all at once or too many contradictory opinions."
3. "When confidential information is shared with two therapists, the risks of breaking confidence may be higher."
4. Especially disconcerting for therapists can be the inappropriate disclosure of personal information about your co-therapist during the session. This can result in a lack of trust between therapists and must be promptly confronted *outside* the session. The untrusting co-therapy relationship proves a detriment to clients.
5. It is possible that a co-therapist may attempt literally to steal a patient away from his or her therapist or steal that patient's affection. Stealing the patient is an economic issue and touches on unethical behavior. Stealing affection is a countertransference issue and touches on sibling rivalry for love.

In our interpretation of responses to question 15, we assumed that the principal benefits of co-therapy were related directly to the reasons clinicians chose the practice of co-therapy. We report in detail on each of these felicitous consequences in Chapter 1. The benefits cited by our sample fall into 13 categories and are listed below along with the number of therapists who specified each.

| Benefit | Frequency of response |
|---|---|
| Greater opportunity for learning through discussion and collaboration with a co-therapist | 25 |
| Widened perspectives for a co-therapist | 25 |
| Widened transference possibilities for patients | 22 |
| Greater learning opportunities for patients | 19 |
| Allows therapists to check and balance their complementary behavior | 19 |
| Synergy | 15 |
| Greater support for therapists and patients | 13 |
| Role flexibility | 10 |
| Share work and responsiblity with co-therapist | 9 |
| Joy, excitement and stimulation for therapists | 6 |
| Greater awareness of counter-transference and enmeshment | 6 |
| Economy of time | 3 |
| Softens the tyranny of one | 2 |

## EXAMPLE OF A CONTRACT BETWEEN NEQUIPOS

A supervisor and a student or a therapist and an assistant therapist who undertake a mode of therapy together we call nequipos. The following is an example of a contract for nequipos, in which the assistant therapist is also an intern.

1. This contract constitutes the agreement between _____ , hereinafter called the therapist and _____ , hereinafter called the intern.
2. The therapist and the intern agree to establish a nequipo team for a period of one year with the understanding that their collaboration may be extended upon mutual agreement of both parties.
3. As nequipos, the therapist and intern propose to co-lead family and group therapy sessions for _____ hours each week. More or less collaboration time can be negotiated if mutually agreeable to both parties. In addition the therapist commits to _____ hour(s) of supervision each week with the intern. The supervisory sessions are in partial fulfillment of the intern's requirements for licensure in the state of  . (In an organization the supervisory sessions are in keeping with the terms of the assistant therapist's job description as an employee at the following institution: _____ .) In these supervisory sessions, the nequipos will review and discuss not only the content of treatment sessions, but also the progress of their work relationship.
4. Following the laws of the state of _____ , the intern will (pay, not pay) for hours of supervision. The intern will (receive, not receive) payment for his or her work as co-leader. The therapist will profit from the collaboration in the following way: . (In an organization where the assistant therapist is an employee, he or she shall receive his or her supervision during paid work time. The therapist will be paid for supervising as part of his or her salary and according to his or her job description.)
5. The therapist's goals for the intern are as follows: _____
6. The intern's goals specific to the nequipo training are as follows: ___
   _____
7. As the assistant therapist in a nequipo team, the intern understands that he or she does not share equal responsibility for the family or group and will not share equally in compensation.
8. The intern's responsibilities shall include but not necessarily be limited to the following functions: in the company of the therapist, he or she will interview prospective families or couples for treatment and will interview prospective group members and assist in their selection for group; he or she will participate in various leadership tasks appropriate to his or her level of clinical skill; he or she will assume greater clinical responsibility as the relationship between the nequipos matures; (add other responsibilities as appropriate).
9. When the therapist plans to be absent from a family or group session, the intern will lead it alone and the therapist will provide supervision and coverage during the treatment session. In the event the therapist

is absent from the treatment site, the therapist will provide at his or her own expense (or at the expense of the organization, if so employed) alternate supervision and coverage during the treatment session.

10. If the terms of this contract prove unsatisfactory to either party, third party consultation will be considered as an option to termination and the therapist will pay if there is any cost. If the nequipos are employees of an organization, third party consultation will be provided at the organization's expense by the following individual: _____ .

This contract may be terminated at any time upon the mutual agreement of both parties giving proper consideration to the need of families and groups in treatment to terminate from their nequipo team.

## EXAMPLE OF A CONTRACT BETWEEN A SUPERVISOR AND CO-LEARNERS

Two students who undertake a mode of therapy together under the aegis of a supervisor we call co-learners. The following is an example of a contract between two co-learners and their supervisor.

1. This contract constitutes the agreement between _____, hereinafter called the supervisor, and _____ and hereinafter called the co-learners.
2. The co-learners agree to establish a co-learner team for a period of nine months and the supervisor agrees to oversee their clinical work and professional relationship during that period. The collaboration between co-learners may be extended upon mutual agreement of all parties, providing that adequate supervision is continued.
3. The co-learners propose to co-lead family and group therapy sessions for _____ hours each week. More or less collaboration time can be negotiated if mutually agreeable to both parties. In addition the supervisor commits to _____ hour(s) of supervision each week with the co-learners. The supervisory sessions are in partial fulfillment of the co-learners' requirements for licensure in the state of _____ . (In an organization the supervisory sessions are in keeping with the terms of the co-learners' job description and the supervisor's job description as employees at the following institution: _____ .) In these supervisory sessions, the co-learners will review and discuss not only the content of treatment sessions, but also the progress of their work relationship.
4. Following the laws of the state of _____ , the co-learners shall (pay, not pay) for hours of supervision. The co-learners will (receive, not receive) payment for their work as co-leaders. The supervisor will profit from the collaboration in the following way: _____ (In an organization: the co-learners shall receive their supervision during paid work time. The supervisor will be paid for his oversight as part of his or her salary and according to his or her job description.)
5. The supervisor's goals for the co-learners are as follows: _____ _____ _____ .
6. The co-learners' goals specific to the co-learner training or experience are as follows: _____ _____ _____ .
7. The co-learners understand that although they share as partners equal responsibility for the families or groups they will co-lead, full clinical responsibility for the course of treatment rests with the supervisor.
8. The co-learners' responsibilities may include but not necessarily be limited to the following functions: whenever possible, co-learners will interview prospective families or couples for treatment and will interview prospective group members and assist in their selection for

group; they will participate in various leadership tasks appropriate to their level of clinical skill; they will assume greater clinical responsibility as the relationship between them matures and at such time when the supervisor judges them ready; (add other responsibilities as appropriate).

9. When one member of the co-learner pair plans to be absent from a family or group treatment session, the other co-learner will lead it alone and supervision will occur at the regularly appointed time. In the event the supervisor is absent from the treatment site, the supervisor will provide at his or her own expense (or at the expense of the organization, if so employed) alternate supervision and coverage during the treatment session.

10. If the terms of this contract prove unsatisfactory to either co-learners or their supervisor, the following individual is deemed suitable as a consultant for conflict resolution as an option to termination of the contract _____ . This contract may be terminated at any time upon the mutual agreement of all parties giving proper consideration to the need of families and groups in treatment to terminate from their co-learner team.

## TABLES

### TABLE A. The Phases of Group Development
### (By Ariadne P. Beck)

| | |
|---|---|
| Phase I | The focus of Phase I is on the creation of a contract to become a working group, based on an initial assessment of the members and an initial statement of goals. |
| Phase II | Phase II has the primary tasks of forging a group identity, clarifying long-term goals, formulating an initial set of norms for functioning in the group, selecting the leaders, and managing the negative emotions that are generated by the competitive work style of this period. All of this must be resolved before the group can move on. |
| Phase III | Phase III is the first cooperative work phase in which members disclose themselves and further define personal goals. Here there is experimentation with a work style for the group. A basic peer equality is established in this phase. |
| Phase IV | During Phase IV, a positive peer bond is formed via the exploration of closeness in the group and discussion about close relationships outside of the group. |
| Phase V | This is followed in Phase V by an exploration of the implications of intimacy, particularly for independency and independency issues among the group members and leader(s). Mutuality and reciprocity are established in an operational way. |
| Phase VI | The members are now free to move forward on the basis of a commitment to each other and the task leader is integrated into the group during Phase VI. |
| Phase VII | Members pursue in-depth self-confrontation of their most basic (sometimes primitive) issues in a safe, supportive, interdependent context in which formal and informal roles have dissipated, replaced by flexible responses based on an in-the-moment assessment of needs and readiness to respond. |
| Phase VIII | When a group knows it will end, Phase VIII deals with an evaluation or review of what has been accomplished and learned, with a focus on the transfer of learning to the rest of one's life. |
| Phase IX | Termination raises the problem for the members of coping with the acknowledgement of their significance to each other while dealing with separation and loss. |

**TABLE B. Emerging Leaders**[a]
**(By Ariadne P. Beck)**

| Leader | Conflict Modeled | Role Function |
|---|---|---|
| Task | This leader either exercises his or her own power and control or gives and shares power with other members. | Convener; selects members; communication expert; self-exploration expert; influences norms, goals; deals with boundaries of group/context. |
| Emotional | This leader struggles with whether to form deep bonds or deny the need for deep bonds with others and whether to affiliate with or reject others. | Models the change process for the group; is best liked in the group; is motivated to participate in the task; monitors the emotional process in the group; is the most important peer support person in the group. |
| Scapegoat | This leader struggles with aggression/submission issues and with the question of whether to assert the self or conform to the group. | Offers a counterpoint to the group concerning the formation of norms; acts as gatekeeper regarding clarity of issues and explanations; focuses on group-as-a-whole issues. |
| Defiant | This leader struggles with whether to take care of and protect the self or to either mistrust other members or merge with them. | Is ambivalent about membership in group; about the need for independence or dependence on authority; about closeness to peers; about self-disclosure. |

[a]These leadership roles will emerge early in a group's life and evolve over the course of the nine phases of development (Beck et al., 1989).

# References

Adler, A. (1930). *Guiding the child on the principles of individual psychology.* New York: Greenberg.

Alpher, V. S., & Kobos, J. C. (1988). Cotherapy in psychodynamic group psychotherapy: An approach to training. *Group, 12(3)* 135–144.

American Psychiatric Association. (1980). *Diagnostic and statistical manual* (Third Edition). Washington, D.C.

Bach, G.R., & Wyden, P. (1970). *The intimate enemy.* New York: Avon Books.

Barnett, F., & Barnett, S. (1988). *Working together: Entrepreneurial couples.* Berkeley, CA: Ten Speed Press.

Beck, A.P. (1974) Phases in the development of structure in therapy and encounter groups. In D. Wexler & L.N.Rices (Eds.) *Innovations in client-centered therapy* (pp. 421–463). New York: Wiley Interscience.

Beck, A. P. (1981a). Developmental characteristics of the system forming process. In J. Durkin (Ed.), *Living groups: Group psychotherapy and general systems theory* (pp. 316–332). New York: Brunner/Mazel.

Beck, A. P. (1981b). The study of group phase development and emergent leadership. *Group, 5(4)*, 48–54.

Beck, A.P., Dugo, J.M., Eng, A.M.,& Lewis, C.M. (1986). The search for phases in group development: designing process analysis measures of group interaction. In L. S. Greenberg & W. M. Pinsoff (Eds.), *The psychotherapeutic process: A research handbook* (pp. 615–705). New York: Guilford Press.

Beck, A. P.,Eng, A.M., & Brusa, J.A. (1989). The evolution of leadership during group development. *Group, 13(3 & 4)* 155–164.

Beck, A.P., & Peters, L.N. (1981). The research evidence for distributed leadership in therapy groups. *International Journal of Group Psychotherapy, 31(1)*, 43–71.

Benjamin, S.E. (1972). Co-therapy: A growth experience for therapists. *International Journal of Group Psychotherapy, 22*, 199–209.

Bernard, H. S., Babineau, R., & Schwartz, A. J. (1980). Supervisor–trainee co-therapy as a method for individual psychotherapy training, *Psychiatry, 15(2)*, 138–145.

Bernard, H.S., Drob, S. L., & Lifshutz, H. (1987). Compatibility between cotherapists: An empirical report, *Psychotherapy, 24*, 96–104.

Berne, E. (1961). *Transactional analysis in psychotherapy*. New York: Grove Press.

Berne, E. (1964). *Games people play*. New York: Grove Press.

Berne, E. (1972). *What do you say after you say hello?* New York: Grove Press.

Bion, Wilfred. (1959). *Experiences in groups*. New York: Basic Books.

Block, S. (1961). Multi-leadership as a teaching and therapeutic tool in group practice. *Comprehensive Psychiatry, 2*, 211–218.

Brent, D.A., & Marine, E. (1982). Developmental aspects of the co-therapy relationship. *Journal of Marital and Family Therapy, 4*, 69–74.

Burns, J. M. (1978). *Leadership* (p. 18). New York: Harper Torchbooks.

Contreras, R., & Scheingold, L. (1984). Couples groups in family practice training. *The Journal of Family Practice, 18(2)*, 293–296.

Cooper, L. (1976). Co-therapy relationships in groups. *Small Group Behavior, 7(4)*, 473–498.

Davis, F. N., & Lohr, M. (1971). Specific problems in the use of co-therapists in group psychotherapy. *International Journal of Group Psychotherapy, 21*, 143–158.

Dick, B., Lessler, K., & Whiteside, J. (1980). A developmental framework for cotherapy. *International Journal of Group Psychotherapy, 30(3)*, 273–285.

Dies, R. R. (1974). Attitudes toward the training of group psychotherapists. *Small Group Behavior, 5*, 65–79.

Dies, R. R. (1980). Current practice in the training of group psychotherapists. *International Journal of Group Psychotherapy, 30(2)*, 169–185.

Dies, R. R., Mallet, J., & Johnson, F. (1979). Openness in the co-leader relationship. Its effect on group process and outcome. *Small Group Behavior, 10(4)*, 523–545.

Dreikurs, R., Shulman,B. H., & Mosak, H. (1952a). Patient–therapist relationship in multiple psychotherapy. I. Its advantages to the therapist. *PSA Quarterly, 26*, 219–227.

Dugo, J.M., & Beck, A.P. (1985). Phases of development of the co-therapy relationship. Presented at the American Group Psychotherapy Association, New York.

Durkin, J. (Ed.). (1981). *Living groups: Group psychotherapy and general systems theory*. New York: Brunner/Mazel.

Gallogly, V., & Levine, B. (1979). Co-therapy. In *Group psychotherapy: practice and development*. Englewood Cliffs, NJ: Prentice Hall.

Gans, R. W. (1962). Group co-therapists and the therapeutic situation: A critical evaluation. *International Journal of Group Psychotherapy, 12*, 82–88.

Getty, C., & Shannon, A. (1969). Co-therapy as an egalitarian relationship. *American Journal of Nursing, 69*, 767–771.

Golden, J. S., & Golden, M. A. (1976). You know who and what's her name: The woman's role in sex therapy. *Journal of Sex and Marital Therapy, 2(1)*, 6–16.

Goulding, R. L., & Goulding, M. M. (1980). *The power is in the patient* (pp. 19–20). San Francisco: Transactional Analysis Press.

Grinberg, L., Sor, D., & deBianchedi, E.T. (1977). *Introduction to the works of Bion* (p. 29). New York: Jason Aronson.

Hadden, S.B. (1947). The utilization of a therapy group in teaching psychotherapy. *American Journal of Psychiatry, 103*, 644–648.

Hannum, J. W. (1980). Some co-therapy techniques with families. *Family Process, 19(2)*, 161–168.

Heilfron, M. (1969). Co-therapy: The relationship between therapists. *International Journal of Group Psychotherapy, 19(3)*, 366–381.

Hoffman, L. W., & Hoffman, H. J. (1981). Husband and wife co-therapy team: Exploration of its development. *Psychotherapy, Theory, Research and Practice, 18(2)*, 217–224.

Jackson, D.D. (1957a). A note on the genesis of trauma in schizophrenia. *Psychiatry, 20*, 181–184.

Jackson, D.D. (1957b). The psychiatrist in the medical clinic. *Bulletin of the American Association of Medical Clinics, 6*, 94–98.

Jackson, D.D. (1957c). The question of family homeostasis. *Psychiatric Quarterly Supplement, 31*, 79–90.

Kahler, T., & Capers, H. (1974). The miniscript. *Transactional Analysis Journal, 4(1)*, 26–42.

Karpman, S. B. (1968). Fairy tales and script drama analysis. *Transactional Analysis Bulletin, 7(26)*, 39–43.

Kernberg, O. (1975). *Borderline conditions and pathological narcissism*. New York: Science House.

Kernberg, O. (1980). *Internal world and external reality: Object relations theory applied*. New York: Jason Aronson.

Kosch, S. G., & Reiner, C. A. (1983). Multiple versus individual therapy: Are two better than one? *American Journal of Psychotherapy, 37(4)*, 567–581.

Langs, R. (1976). *The therapeutic interaction*. New York: Jason Aronson.

LoPiccolo, J., Heiman, J. R., Hogan, D. R., & Roberts, C. W. (1985). Effectiveness of single therapist versus co-therapy teams in sex therapy. *Journal of Consulting and Clinical Psychology, 53(3)*, 287–294.

Lothstein, L. (1979). Group therapy with gender dysphoric patients. *American Journal of Psychotherapy, 33*, 67–88.

Lundin, W. H., & Aranov, B. M. (1952). The use of co-therapists in group psychotherapy. *Journal of Consulting Psychology. 16*, 76–79.

Luthman, S., & Kirschenbaum, M. (1974). *The dynamic family*. Palo Alto, CA: Science and Behavior Books.

Masters, W. H., & Johnson, V. E. (1970). *Human sexual inadequacy*. Boston: Little, Brown.

Masterson, J. F. (1976). *Psychotherapy of the borderline adult*. New York: Brunner/Mazel.

Masterson, J. F. (1981). *The narcissistic and borderline disorders*. New York: Brunner/Mazel.

Matthews, A. The Poppers and the plains. *The New York Times Magazine, June 24, 1990*, pp. 24–26, 41, 48–49, 53.

McGee, T. F., & Schuman, B. N. (1970). The nature of the co-therapy relationship. *International Journal of Group Psychotherapy, 20(1)*, 25–35.

McMahon, N., & Links, P. S. (1984). Co-therapy: The need for positive pairing. *Canadian Journal of Psychiatry, 29(5)*, 385–389.

Mintz, E. E. (1963). Special values of co-therapists in group psychotherapy. *International Journal of Group Psychotherapy, 13(2)*, 127–132.

Minuchin, S., & Fishman, H. C. (1981). *Family therapy techniques (pp.30–31)*. Cambridge: Harvard University Press.

Minuchin, S., Montalvo, B., Guerney, B., Rossman, B., & Schumer, F. (1967). *Families of the slums*. New York: Basic Books.

Napier, A. Y., & Whitaker, C. A. (1988). *The family crucible*. New York: Perennial Library, Harper & Row.

Ogden, T. H. (1979). On projective identification. *International Journal of Psychoanalysis, 60*, 357–373.

Paulson, I., Burroughs J. C., & Gelb, C. B. (1977) Cotherapy: What is the crux of the relationship? *International Journal of Group Psychotherapy*, 213–224.

Peters, L. N., & Beck, A. P. (1982). Identifying emergent leaders in psychotherapy groups. *Group, 6(1)*, 35–40.

Piper, W. E., Doan, B. D., Edwards, E. M., & Jones, B. D. (1979). Cotherapy behavior, group therapy process, and treatment outcome. *Journal of Consulting and Clinical Psychology, 47(6)*, 1081–1089.

Rabin, H. M. (1967). How does co-therapy compare with regular group therapy? *American Journal of Psychotherapy, 21*, 244–255.

Roller, B. (1984). The group therapist: Stages of professional and personal development. *Small Group Behavior, 15(2)*, 265–269.

Roller, B. (1986). Group therapy marks fiftieth birthday. *Small Group Behavior, 17(4)*, 472–474.

Roller, B., Schnell, C., & Welsch, M. (1982). Organization and development of group psychotherapy programs in health maintenance organizations. In *1982 Group Health Institute Proceedings* Washington, DC: The Group Health Association of America. (p. 125).

Roller, W. L., & Shaskan, D. A. (1982). Patients' perceptions of distance: The same therapist in group therapy compared to individual treatment. *Small Group Behavior, 13(1)*, 117–124.

Roman, M., & Meltzer, B. (1977). Co-therapy: A review of current literature with special reference to therapeutic outcome. *Journal of Sex and Marital Therapy, 3(1)*, 63–77.

Roscoe, J. T. (1969). *Fundamental research statistics for the behavioral sciences*. New York: Holt, Rinehart, & Winston.

Rosenbaum, M. (1977). Group therapy and cotherapy. *International Encyclopedia of Psychiatry, Psychology, Psychoanalysis and Neurology, 5*, 283–288.

Rosenbaum, M. (1983). Co-therapy. In H. I. Kaplan & B. J. Sadock (Eds.), *Comprehensive group psychotherapy* (pp. 167–183). Baltimore: Williams & Wilkins.

Rosenthall, P. (1946). Death of co-therapist. *American Journal of Orthopsychiatry*.

Rubinstein, D., & Weiner, O. R. (1967). Co-therapy teamwork relationships in family psychotherapy. In G. H. Zuk and I. Boszormenyi-Nagy (Eds.), *Family therapy of disturbed families* (pp. 206–220). Palo Alto, CA: Science and Behavioral Books.

Russell, A., & Russell, L. (1979). The uses and abuses of co-therapy. *The Journal of Marital and Family Therapy, 5(1)*, 39–46.

Rutan, J. S., & Stone, W. (1984). *Psychodynamic group psychotherapy.* Lexington, MA: Collamore Press.

Sager, C. J., & Kaplan, H. S. (1972). The marriage contract. In C. J. Sager and H. S. Kaplan (Eds.), *Progress in group and family therapy* (pp. 483–497). New York: Brunner/Mazel.

Satir, V. (1964). *Conjoint family therapy.* Palo Alto, CA: Science and Behavior Books.

Satir, V. (1972). *Peoplemaking.* Palo Alto, CA : Science and Behavior Books.

Schiff, J. L. (1969) Reparenting schizophrenics. *Transactional Analysis Bulletin, 8 (31)*, 47–63.

Schilder, P. (1985). Body image and social psychology. In D. A. Shaskan & W. L. Roller (Eds.), *Paul Schilder: Mind explorer* (pp. 219–229). New York: Human Sciences Press.

Shaskan, D. A., & Roller, W. L. (1985). *Paul Schilder: Mind explorer* (pp. 47–48). New York: Human Sciences Press.

Silber, T.J., & Bogado, P. (1983). Pediatrician and psychiatrist as co-therapists. *Adolescence, 18 (70)*, 331–337.

Snyder, G. (1985). *Axe handles.* San Francisco: North Point Press.

Whitaker, C., & Garfield, R. (1987). On teaching psychotherapy via consultation and cotherapy. *Contemporary Family Therapy, 9(1–2)*, 106–115.

White, E. M. (1986). Sexual attraction between male and female co-leaders of group psychotherapy: Occurrence and effects. Paper presented at the American Group Psychotherapy Association Annual Conference, Washington, D.C.

Williams, R. (1976). A contract for co-therapists in group psychotherapy. *Journal of Psychiatric Nursing, 14(6)*, 11–14.

Winter, S. K. (1976). Developmental stages in the roles and concerns of group co-leaders. *Small Group Behavior, 7(3)*, 349–362.

Yalom, I. D. (1970). *The theory and practice of group psychotherapy* (pp. 318–321). New York: Basic Books.

Zilbergeld, B., & Evans, M. (1980). The inadequacy of Masters and Johnson. *Psychology Today, 14*, 29–43.

♦ ♦

# Suggested Further Readings

Andersen, T. (1987). The general practitioner and consulting psychiatrist as a team with "stuck" families. *Family Systems Medicine, 5(4)*, 468–481.

Barnard, C.P., & Miller, B. (1987). Cotherapy: A means of training with the family, *Australian and New Zealand Journal of Family Therapy, 8(3)*, 137–142.

Bateson, G. (1972). *Steps to an ecology of mind.* San Francisco: Chandler.

Beck, R. L., & Bosman-Clark, J. (1989). The written summary in group psychotherapy revisited. *Group, 13(2)*, 102–111.

Bellville, T. P., Raths, O. N., & Bellville, C. J. (1969). Conjoint marriage therapy with a husband-and-wife team, *American Journal of Orthopsychiatry, 39*, 473–483.

Bowers, W.A., & Gauron, E. F. (1981). Potential hazards of the co-therapy relationship, *Psychotherapy: Theory, Research and Practice, 18(2)*, 225–228.

Briggs, J. P., & Briggs, M. A. (1979). Treating the marital crisis with the two-marriage equation, *Journal of Sex and Marital Therapy, 5(1)*, 28–40.

Canino, G., & Canino I.A. (1982). Culturally syntonic family therapy for migrant Puerto Ricans. *Hospital and Community Psychiatry, 33(4)*, 299–303.

Cornwell, M., & Pearson, R. (1981). Cotherapy teams and one-way screen in family therapy practice and training. *Family Process, 20(2)*, 199–209.

del Pino Perez, Antonio. (1981). Cotherapists in educational behavior therapy: Evaluation of an intervention strategy. *Analisis y Modificacion de Conducta, 7(16)*, 127–176.

Demarest, E. W., & Teicher, A. (1954). Transference in group therapy: Its use by co-therapists of opposite sexes. *Psychiatry, 17*, 187–202.

Douglas, A. R., & Matson, I. C. (1989). An account of a time-limited therapeutic group in an NHS setting women with a history of incest. *Group, 13(2)*, 83–94.

Dreikurs, R. (1950). Techniques and dynamics of multiple psycho-therapy. *Psychiatric Quarterly, 24*, 788–799

Dreikurs, R., Shulman, B. H., & Mosak, H. (1952b). Patient-therapist relationship in multiple psychotherapy. II Its advantages for the patient. *PSA Quarterly, 26,* 590–596.

Farhood, L. (1975). Choosing a partner for co-therapy. *Perspectives in Psychiatric Care, 13(4),* 177–179.

Fong, J. Y., Schneider, M., & Walls-Cooke, P. (1978). Multiple family group therapy with a tri-therapist team. *Nursing Clinics of North America, 13(4),* 685–699.

Gans, R. W. (1957). The use of group co-therapists in the teaching of psychotherapy. *American Journal of Psychotherapy, 11,* 618–625.

Gonzalez, J. L., Diaz de Mathmann, C., & Doring, R. (1982). Co-therapy in a group of lower class psychosomatic patients. *Dynamische Psychiatrie, 15(1-2),* 21–33.

Greenblum, D. N., & Pinney, E. L. (1982). Some comments on the role of cotherapists in group psychotherapy with borderline patients. *Group, 6(1),* 41–47.

Haber, R., & Cooper-Haber, K. (1987). Paradox and orthodox: A cotherapy approach. *Journal of Strategic and Systemic Therapies. 6(2),* 41–50.

Hafner, R. J. (1981). "Spouse-aided therapy in psychiatry: An introduction. *Australian and New Zealand Journal of Psychiatry, 15(4),* 329–337.

Haley, J. (1976). *Problem solving therapy.* San Francisco: Jossey–Bass.

Heijkoop, J. (1982). A unique information source in mediation therapy. *Gedragstherapie, 15(1),* 58–64.

Hellwig, K., & Memmott, R. J. (1974). Co-therapy: The balancing act. *Small Group Behavior, 5(2),* 175–181.

Hellwig, K., & Memmott, R. J. (1978). Partners in therapy: Using the co-therapists' relationship in a group. *Journal of Psychiatric Nursing, 16(4),* 41–44.

Hoffman, S., Kohener, R., & Shapira, M. (1987). Two on one: Dialectical psychotherapy. *Psychotherapy, 24(2),* 212–216.

Hoffman, S., & Merdler, A. (1988). Use of dialectical psychotherapy in treating bulimarexic disorders: A case study. *Journal of Contemporary Psychotherapy, 18(3),* 217–225.

Holt, M., & Greiner, D. (1976). Co-Therapy in the treatment of families. In P. J. Guerin, Jr. (Ed.), *Family therapy: theory and practice.* New York: Gardner Press.

Hulse, W. C., Lulow, W. V., Rindsberg, P.S.W., & Epstein, N.B. (1956). Transference reactions in a group of female patients to male and female co-leaders. *International Journal of Group Psychotherapy, 6(4),* 430–435.

Kennedy, J. F. (1989). Therapist gender and the same-sex puberty age psychotherapy group. *International Journal of Group Psychotherapy, 39(2),* 255–263.

Lazarus, L. W. (1976). Family therapy by a husband–wife team. *Journal of Marriage and Family Counseling, 25,* 225–233.

Levin, P. (1974). *Becoming the way we are.* Sacramento, CA: Jalmar Press.

Levine, C. O., & Dang, J. C. (1979). The group within the group: The dilemna of co-therapy. *International Journal of Group Psychotherapy, 29(2),* 175–184.

Lothstein, L. (1980). Co-therapy and supervision. In Wolberg and Aronson (Eds.), *Group and family therapy.* New York: Brunner/Mazel.

MacLennan, B. W. (1965). Co-therapy. *International Journal of Group Psychotherapy, 15*, 154–166.

Mathews, A., Whitehead, A., & Kellett, J. M. (1983). Psychological and hormonal factors in the treatment of female sexual dysfunction. *Psychological Medicine, 13(1)*, 83–92.

McGee, T. F. (1974). The triadic approach to supervision in group psychotherapy. *International Journal of Group Psychotherapy, 24*, 471–475.

Mehlman, S. K., Baucom, D. H., & Anderson, D. (1983). Effectiveness of cotherapists versus single therapists and immediate versus delayed treatment in behavioral marital therapy. *Journal of Consulting and Clinical Psychology, 51(2)*, 258–266.

Meyerstein, I., & Kompass, F. R. (1987). Teaching the mechanics of design, collaboration, and delivery of the final intervention in a team based live supervision group. *Journal of Strategic and Systemic Therapies. 6(1)*, 39–51.

Mintz, E. E. (1965). Male–female co-therapists: Some values and some problems. *American Journal of Psychotherapy, 19*, 293–301.

Obler, M. (1982). A comparison of hypnoanalytic/behavior modification technique and a cotherapist-type treatment with primary orgasmic dysfunction females: Some preliminary results. *Journal of Sex Research, 18(1)*, 331–345.

Oldham, J. M. (1982). The use of silent observers as an adjunct to short-term inpatient group psychotherapy. *International Journal of Group Psychotherapy, 32(4)*, 169–180.

Ormont, L. R. (1981). Principles and practice of conjoint psychoanalytic treatment. *American Journal of Psychiatry, 138(1)*, 69–73.

Palandjian, G. E. (1982). Games and child co-therapies. *Neuropsychiatrie de l'Enfance et de l'Adolescence, 30(7–8)*, 441–444.

Perls, F. S. (1969). *Gestalt therapy verbatim.* New York: Bantam Books.

Petrovic, D., & Sedmak, T.(1982). Education in the large group. *Psihijatrija Danas, 14(1)*, 39–44.

Pfeiffer, J. W., & Jones, J. E. (1975). Co-facilitating. *Annual Handbook for Group Facilitators*, 219–227.

Pietz, C. A., & Mann, J. P. (1989). Importance of having a female therapist in a child molesters' group. *Professional Psychology: Research and Practice, 20(4)*, 265–268.

Popovic, M. (1982). The meeting of the therapeutic team after the large group. *Psihijatrija Danas, 14(1)*, 136–138.

Rabin, C., Rosenbaum, H., & Sens, M. (1982). Home-based marital therapy for multiproblem families. *Journal of Marital and Family Therapy, 8(1)*, 151–161.

Reynolds, B. S., Cohen, B. D., Schochet, B. V., Price, S. C., & Anderson, A. J. (1981) Dating skills training in the group treatment of erectile dysfunction for men without partners. *Journal of Sex and Marital Therapy, 7(3)*, 184–194.

Rickarby, G., & Egan, P. (1981). Family therapy in the playroom. *International Journal of Family Psychiatry, 2(3–4)*, 221–235.

Roller, B., & Lankester, D. (1987). Characteristic processes and therapeutic strategies in a homogeneous group for depressed outpatients. *Small Group Behavior, 18(4)*, 565–576.

Seeman, M. V., Pyke, J., Denberg, D., Blake, P., & Freire, M. (1976). Focus on co-therapy in a rehabilitation programme for advanced schizophrenia. *Canadian Mental Health, 24(3)*, 13–14.

Seeman, M. V., Pyke, J., Denberg, D., Blake, P., & Freire, M. (1982) Co-therapy in a clinic for schizophrenia. *Canadian Journal of Psychiatry, 27(4)*, 296–300.

Smith, L., & Vannicelli, M. (1985). Coleader termination in an outpatient alcohol treatment group. *Group, 9(3)*, 49–56.

Solomon, A., Loeffler, F. J., & Frank, G. H. (1953). An analysis of co-therapist interaction in group psychotherapy. *International Journal of Group Psychotherapy, 3(2)*, 171–180.

Starak, Y. (1981). Co-leadership: A new look at sharing group work. *Social Work with Groups, 4(3–4)*, 145–157.

Stone, M. H. (Ed.), (1986). *Essential papers on borderline disorders: One hundred years at the border.* New York University Press.

Todd, T. C., & Greenberg, A. (1987). No question has a single answer: Integrating discrepant models in family therapy training. *Contemporary Family Therapy, 9(1–2)*, 116–137.

Vannicelli, M. (1987). Treatment of alcoholic couples in outpatient group therapy. *Group, 11(4)*, 247–257.

Warkentin, J., Johnson, N. L., & Whitaker, C. A. (1951). A comparison of individual and multiple psychotherapy. In W. A. White (Ed.), *Psychiatry* (pp.415–418). New York: Psychiatric Foundation.

Waters, C. W., & Pullen, M. (1968). Effect of the sudden departure and replacement of one member of a co-therapy team on a married couples group, *Psychiatric Quarterly, 42*, 65–74.

Whitaker, C., Warkentin, J., & Johnson, N. (1950). The psychotherapeutic impasse. *American Journal of Orthopsychiatry, 20*, 641–647.

# Index

Abuse, sexual
  breakthrough about, and cessation
    of co-therapy, 137
  of children, therapy for, 25, 78–79,
    111
  opposite-sex co-therapists for diag-
    nosis of, 137
Ackerman, Nathan, 218
Acknowledgement of accomplishment, 16, 46–47
Acting out, 18, 57, 58, 59, 116, 125,
  177
Adler, Alfred, 6, 137
Adler, Alexandra, 6
Adolescents, 47–48, 57, 59, 60
  female, entering puberty, 59–60
  male, adult modeling and impulse
    control for, 57
Aggression, 57, 89
Alcoholism in families of origin, 56,
  107
American Group Psychotherapy
  Association, survey of, 1, 11, 200,
  222–228
  assets and qualities sought for rela-
    tionship, 226
  disinterest in co-therapy, 225
  questionnaire, 223–224
  sample, 222, 224–225
  sex preferred in co-therapist,
    226–227
  trainees, use of, 227–228

Anger, 109, 113, 145, 146
Anxiety, 21, 27, 47, 76, 82, 108–110,
  115, 117, 138, 149, 166
Appreciation from other co-therapist,
  importance of, 194
Assertiveness, therapeutic, 43, 45, 50,
  60, 100, 127, 129
Assignment to partner vs. autonomy
  in choice, 62–63
Assistant therapists; *see also* Nequipos
  acknowledgement of, 46–47
  co-leading with a supervisor, 200
  honesty about in therapy, 200–201

## B

Backups, co-therapists as, 25, 208
Balancing principle, 3, 66, 121
Bateson, Gregory, 218
"Be Perfect" driver, 119–120, 230
Beck, Ariadne, 5, 30, 31, 33, 81, 85,
  96, 98, 101, 103
  group therapy process research of,
    156, 236–237
Bion, work of, 134, 141
Body image, 23
Body work, 148
Bonding, of patients with therapists,
  13–14; *see also* Co-therapists
  group issues
  questions for co-therapists, 14
  transference by patients, 13

Borderline personality, 49, 107–108
  Christine's case; *see also* Counter-
    transference
  body boundary, 136, 137
  boundaries in, 132
  diagnostic criteria, 131–133
  dreams, 132
  group therapy of, 136
  men, relationships with, 136
  negative transference, 136
  others, attitudes to, 132
  projections by, 135, 136
  protection of from abuse memo-
    ries, 135
  psychic experiences, 132
  rage of, 132
  recapitulation of family experi-
    ence, 137
  regression, 136–137
  and reparenting, 139
  resistance of, 133
  self, attitudes to, 132
  self-representation of, 131
  sexual abuse of during childhood,
    135, 136, 137
  splitting of between therapists,
    135
  strategy for treatment, 132–133
  strengths and weaknesses, 132
Boundaries, 53, 76, 111, 123, 127,
    136, 148, 150, 181
  of body, 136, 137
  with client, 123
  between co-therapists, 73–74
  establishment of, 53, 122–123
  need for maintenance of, 150
  present/past, 136
  reparenting, 139
  in supervisor role, 54
  violation of, 127
Bowen, Murray, 218
Burnout, 16
Burns, James MacGregor, 4
Business, co-leadership in, 4–5

C

Change, resistance to, 221
Child abuse, 211
Clarity
  need for, 112–114, 213
  personal, 2–3
Clients as "co-therapists," 201

Clinical decisions, sharing in, 86, 103,
    116
Co-dependency, 60–61, 88–90,
    117–121, 126, 128
  between co-learners, 60–61
  between co-therapists, 107,
    117–121
    avoidance of mentioning
      co-dependency, 118–119
    countertransference in family
      therapy, 119
    denial of, 119
    fears of solo work, 118
    of couple, 88, 107
Co-learners
  co-dependency between, 60–61
  countertransference in, 55–56
  defined, 38
  learning contract for, 44–46
  as research subjects, 40
  risks inherent to training of, 45
  rules for supervisors of, 42–43
  supervision of, 41–43
  termination procedures for, 45
Collusion, 108–114, 126
  against group by co-therapists, 109
  anger, problems with, 108–109
  avoidance of, 146
  by one therapist against another, 110
  clarity, lack of, 112
  communication problems, 112–114
  consultation about, 108
  fears of co-therapists, 109
  inability to handle group, case, 113
  with group by co-therapists during
    scapegoating, 108–109
Commitment
  of nequipos, 43, 44, 52–53
  of supervisors, 40, 43, 52–53
  of therapists, 3, 32, 44, 64, 125
Competence
  definition of, 67
  desire to project as assistant thera-
    pist, 49
  vs. perfectionism, realism about, 120
Competition, 100–106, 156, 172–173,
    193
  between therapists vs. equality, 84
  for client, 102
  control of, 64
  dialogue about, 101
  healthy vs. unhealthy, 100
  and humor, 103

for importance in patients' lives,
102
"ownership" of client, 102
for praise of supervisor, 58–59
rivalry, signs of, 102–103
with supervisor, 57–58
unrecognized, 121
Complementarity, 27–29
and equality, 27–28
of personal attributes and skills,
28–29
Conflicts between co-therapists,
103–106; *see also* Disagreements
Confrontation, 57, 59, 80, 132–133
Congruence
between co-therapists, 114–117,
220
and co-therapy, 74, 114–117
definition of, 211
double bind on patient, 114, 115
lack of leads to group termination,
116
and wedge driven between therapists by patient, 115
Consultation
between co-therapists, 16, 90, 103
with co-therapists, 85, 96, 105–106,
108, 117, 126, 128
with nequipos, 48, 50
with a peer group, 123
Contract
between co-leaders, 163
between co-learners, 44–46
betwen nequipos, 43–44
between therapist and patient, 133,
151, 215
co-therapy, 73–74
Co-therapists
commitment of, 4
compatibility of viewpoints,
77–79
death of, 63
flexibility in roles, 20–21
games of, 205
group issues, 162
bonding, 165, 167–168, 170,
174–175, 177, 179, 181–182,
184, 186
compatibility, 164–165, 167, 169,
174, 177, 179, 181, 184, 186,
195–197
stresses, 165, 170, 175, 177–178,
179, 182, 184–186

homosexual, 48, 126
open sexual involvement of, 32–35
personal problems of, 196, 215
qualities desired in by therapists,
63–65
relationship issues, 162
attraction, 146, 163, 165–166,
168, 173, 175, 178, 180, 182,
185
communication, 164, 166–167,
169, 173–174, 176, 178–179,
181, 183, 185–186
gains, 163–164, 166, 168, 173,
175–176, 178, 180, 182–183,
185
negotiation, 164, 166–167, 169,
173–174, 176, 178–179, 181,
183, 185–186
secret sexual involvement of,
125–128
self-selective process in selection of,
67
sexual attraction between, 31–32
in supervision, 98–100
their willingness to reveal themselves, 85
theoretical orientations of, 12–13,
77–79
therapeutic identity of, 186
unequal, problems with, 35–36
Co-therapy
advantages of, 206–208
atmosphere of, 20
benefits of, 15–21, 231
choice of partners, Satir's questions,
220–221
choice of relationship by therapists,
12
with a co-dependent couple, 76
congruence in, 74, 114–117
contract, 73–74
and couples, self-treatment of, 124
definitions, 2, 11
denial of treatment to inappropriate
patient, 25–26
difficulties with, 216–218
equality of therapists, effects on
therapy, 23
factors in success of, 228–230
formal vs. informal aspects of relationship, 161
guidelines for couples who practice,
124–125

guidelines for institutions or group
    private practices, 170–172
hazards to, 97, 230–231
increased costs of, 26
in individual mode, 130, 151
integration of skills in, 199
as means of starting the healing,
    218–219
modes of treatment found in, 130
nature of, 2–4
as peer relationship, 2–3
program, making guidelines for,
    171–172
reasons for, 12, 13, 14, 194
as relationship between
    co-therapists, 3, 11–12
scheduling problems, 27
supervision of, case, 99–100
synergism in, 21
teams, formation of, 63
time requirements for learning of,
    44–45
time, use of, 26
as training for psychotherapy, 37
Co-therapy relationship, benefits to
    therapists
acknowledgements, mutual, 16
companionship, 16
countertransference, dealing with,
    17–19
emotional support for practitioners,
    16–17
mutual assistance of, 20–21
objectivity, 18
one therapist, limits of, 20
primary bond of therapists, 15
reinforcements, 16
role flexibility, 20–21
therapeutic approach, flexibility of,
    21
Co-therapy research, 6–7, 37, 40–41,
    62
of phases of team development,
    155–188
Co-therapy teams
consequences of conflicting mes-
    sages from leaders of, 157
development phases, nine-phase
    theory of, 157–159, 161
dysfunction of, 14, 78, 85–86,
    96–98, 105–106, 109–110,
    111, 124
experience of therapists, differences
    in, 187

identity of team, establishment of,
    172–179
task leadership role, 163
theories about development, com-
    parison, 160
Countertransference, 16, 18, 55–56,
    77–80, 90–91, 106–112, 119,
    133–134, 140–141, 142, 143,
    146–147
awareness of, 133–134
borderline personalities, 80,
    107–108
in burnout, 16
in co-learner teams, 55–56
confrontations between
    co-therapists, 79–80
examples, 79–80
family dynamics, acting out, of, 107
identification of, by co-therapist,
    106–107
prevention of acting out, 90–91
projection onto patient, 108
scapegoating, 108
sex therapy, 107
of supervisor, 59–60
Countertransference, with a border-
    line patient
in co-therapy, 140, 142, 143
co-therapist's help with, 140–141
in response to patient's dissociation,
    142–143


D

Death of co-therapist, 63
Denial, 48–49, 55, 107, 128,
    137–138
breaking through of, 128, 137–138
collusion with, 48–49
of destructive behavior of
    co-therapist, 119
Dependency
of clients, 19, 135
in early phases of co-therapy team
    development, 31
in nequipo teams, 118
Direction shift in therapy, preparation
    for, 112–113
Disagreements
between co-therapists, 23, 78, 111,
    194–195, 217
clients' fears about, 209
vs. disparagement, 103

Dissociation from self, 142–143
Diversion of attention from patients to
   co-therapists, 111
Division of labor, 84, 215
"Divorce" of co-therapists, 205, 206
"Don't be you" injunction, 148
"Don't grow up" injunction, 82
"Don't make it" injunction, 82
Double bind, 114, 115, 148, 218
Dreams
   of co-therapists, 122–123
   of nequipos, 49, 53
   of patients, 114, 122, 132, 137, 139,
   149
Dreikurs, Rudolf, 20
Dual transference, 14, 133
Dugo, James, 5, 30, 31, 81, 96, 101,
   103, 155
Dysfunctional family roles, adoption
   of by co-therapists, 107,
   111–112; *see also* Counter-
   transference

E

Economy in co-therapy, 24–27
Ego, 132–133, 134, 138, 144,
   149–150
Ego states, 149, 194, 197
   child vs. parent, 194
Emerging leaders, roles of, by Ariadne
   P. Beck, 237
Empathy, 60, 65, 132, 143, 148, 149
Enmeshment, 17, 18, 107
Equality, 2, 28, 64, 84–86, 120,
   212–213
   clinical decisions, 86
   competition between co-therapists,
   84
   in co-therapists, 28
   in co-therapy relationship, 212,
   213
   division of labor, 84
   failure to correct misstatements,
   85–86
   family therapy, 84–85, 120–121
   group therapy, phases of, 85
   initial interviews with patients, 85
   lack of, effects, 120–121
   mutual stroking, 86
   prohibition of, in co-therapy pair,
   120
Exclusion of co-therapist, 110

F

Falling in love with patient, 122–123
Family, co-therapy for
   grief of stepmother, 94–95
   loneliness of son, 94
   sorrow of family, 93–94
   therapeutic leverage in, 18–19
   war traumas of father, 93–94
Family, enmeshment and manipulation by, 17–18
Frey, Bill, 218

G

Games, playing of, between
   co-therapists, 205–206
   "If It Weren't for Her or Him,"
   205–206
   "If It Weren't for You," 110
   "Nag Me," 205
Gestalt therapy, 189, 193, 198
Gifts, sharing of, in co-therapy, 67,
   196
Goulding, Robert and Mary, 5, 81,
   82, 87, 104, 120, 121, 122,
   189–209
   clients, conflicts about, 195
   co-therapy, reasons for, 194
   friendships with patients, 193
   team, establishment of, 193
Group-as-a-whole, 78, 108–109, 115,
   116, 145, 157, 165, 166, 167,
   175, 177, 181, 183, 184
   projections onto, 145
Group development phases, 236
Group Health Cooperative of Puget
   Sound, 16, 26, 222
Group process, 55, 77, 78, 156, 165,
   204–205
Group therapy
   asking a patient to leave, 26
   disagreements between
   co-therapists, 115–116
   first co-therapy in hospital, for
   adults, 6
   nequipos' introduction into, 49
   phases of co-therapy team development in, 155–188
   short-term, 187
   supervision of, co-learner team,
   53
   training in, nequipo team, 52

**H**

Haley, Jay, 218
Healing process with two people, co-
    therapy as, 218–219
Honesty, failure of, in co-therapists,
    205
Humor
    in a co-therapy team, 194
    inappropriate, 103
    use of, 76–77

**I**

Impasses, 105–106, 112, 156, 228
    between co-therapists as block to
        therapy, 106
    passive–aggressive, 105
    patient's observation about, 106
    use of second therapist in individual
        hour with client, 228
Impotence, 34, 107
Incentives for group therapy, 16
Incongruence, 116, 141
Individual treatment, 20, 130, 151
Inequality, 35–36, 100
    belief in of therapists, 85
    in nequipo teams, 38, 113
Inflexibility in co-therapists, 112
Interviews
    diagnostic value of, 19
    initial, 8
Intimacy in co-therapists, 29, 30, 31,
    32, 33; *see also entries under* Sexual
    relationship of co-therapists
Isomorphy, 155–156

**J**

Jackson, Don, 218
Jealousy, 121, 122, 123

**K**

Kernberg, Otto, 131, 134
Kirschenbaum, Marty, 17

**L**

Laughter as disparaging message,
    105–106
Leadership, defined, 4
Learning contract for nequipos
    contents of, 43

example of, 232, 233
    scapegoating, 45
    time commitment, 44
Learning contract for supervisors and
    co-learners
    benefits for supervisor, disclosure
        of, 45–46
    competition between co-learners,
        44–45
    content of, 44–46
    example of, 234–235
    mistakes, co-learners' fear of, 45
    partner, choice of, 45
    relationships between co-learners,
        44
    supervisory sessions, length of, 46
    termination procedures, 45–46
    time commitment, 45
Learning model, co-therapy as, 12–13
Learning therapy as, 211
Life script, concept of, 77
Liking, effects of, 87
Listening in group therapy,
    Gouldings' views on, 204
Loneliness, professional, 16, 215
Loss, feelings of with termination,
    15–16
Luthman, Shirley, 17

**M**

Males
    men's groups, 213
    role modeling for, 198, 199
Manipulation by family in therapy,
    17–18
Manipulation by patients, 80, 103,
    108, 142–143
Marriage partners and lovers as co-
    therapists, problems of; *see also*
    *entries under* Co-therapists;
    Co-therapy; Seduction; Sexual
    relationship of co-therapists
    clients, sexual attraction of, to co-
        therapist, 122
    inequality in marriage, 123
    strains on marriage, case, 121
Married couple, co-therapy treatment
    for
    co-dependency, 88
    countertransference, working
        through, 90–91
    defensive postures, breakdown of,
        89

loneliness of husband, 90
modeling of communication, 90
pathological communication cycle, 88
personality differences, work on, 89
rejection, dealing with, 91
Masterson, James, 131
Medication
  decision to prescribe, 104
  disagreements about, 116
Mimicking of client's behavior by co-therapists, 123–124
Mintz, Elizabeth, 14, 135, 151
Minuchin, Salvador, 18
Mirroring of client, 211
Mistakes
  by co-learners, 45, 61, 119–120
  by co-therapists, 25, 85, 97, 126, 130, 140, 148, 196, 215–216
  by nequipos, 35, 48–49
  in psychotherapy, 204, 217
  sharing of, by supervisor, 61
  by trainees, 41
  willing to admit, by co-therapists, 66
Mode of treatment and equality of participation, 84–85
Models and modeling; *see also entries under* Co-therapists; Co-therapy; Therapists as models
  communication between equals, 23
  and creativity, 22
  for human growth, 21–24
  husband and wife team, 215
  nonverbal actions, 23
  open disagreement, 23
  and parenting, parallel to, 22
  transference of qualities to patients, 21–22
  of variety of behavior patterns, 19

N

Napier, Augustus, 3, 21
Narcissistic personality, Kevin's case; *see also* Countertransference
  behavior, changes in, 149
  body therapy for, 148–149
  criticism of group by, 145–146
  devaluation of group, countertransference about, 146
  devaluation of therapy by patient, 146–147

diagnostic criteria, 131–133
distant-and-friendly-mother strategy, 150–151
father, attitudes to, 147, 148
and group therapy, 147–149
hospitalization of, 147
identification with mother, 131
leaving of group, 145
mother, obession about, 145, 146, 147–148
others, attitudes to, 132
positive double bind strategy, 148
rage of, 132
reparenting of, 149–151
as scapegoat, 145, 146
self-representation, 131
strength and weakness in, 132
therapeutic alliance, 148
treatment strategy, 132–133
Narcissistic therapist, 121
Nequipos; *see also* Learning contract for nequipos; Training and trainees
  becoming co-therapists, 52
  commitment of, 39
  defined, 38
  learning contracts, 43, 44, 232–233
  risks inherent to training, 43
  team posing as co-therapists, 118
  unacknowledged team, 47
  unequal status of denied, patients' reactions, 113
Nequipos, teams of
  acknowledgement of assistant therapist, 46–47
  denial by patient, collusion with, 48–49
  difficulties in early stages, 49
  rules for, 42
  seductive assistant therapist, 47–48
  student member of, 187
No-change contract, nonverbal, between patients and co-therapists, 97
"No-secrets" policy between co-therapists, 111
Noise in group life, 156
Non-therapist spouses, feeling excluded, 124
Norms of group, 184, 185
Northern California Group Psychotherapy Society, 1
Novice, apprehension of, 50–51

**O**

Objectivity, mutual provision of, 216
One-upsmanship, 104
Open communication, 79–84
  assumptions of co-therapists, checking of, 81
  countertransference, 79–80
  family therapy, 80–81
  group therapy, 80–82
  instructions between co-therapists, 82
  post-group sessions, 82–84
  signals between co-therapists, 81
  strokes, 81–83
Orientation, theoretical, of therapists; *see* Co-therapists, theoretical orientations of
Out-of-body experiences, 107, 132
Overinvolvement with co-therapist, 27
"Ownership" of clients, 102, 182

**P**

Paradoxical intent strategy, 120
Parent objects, therapists as, 14
Parents and parenting; *See also entries under* Co-therapy; Reparenting
  and co-therapy, 4, 14, 21–24, 135–137, 206, 210
  as earliest people child sees, 22–23
  and modeling, 22
  and triads, 219–220
Passive–aggressive problem, 104–105, 205–206
Peer consultation relationship, 180
Performance anxiety, 120
Personal information, inappropriate disclosure of, 231
Personal problems of co-therapists, 196–197
Physician/nonphysician pairs, 116
Post-session work, 50, 51, 142
Power struggles, 34–35, 103, 176, 185
  between co-therapists, 103
  decision making, 103
  in married couples, 34–35
Power to make known, 35
Primary process, 132, 138
Private understandings with patients, 111

Projection
  onto group, 145
  onto patients, problems with, 108
Projective identification
  awareness of, 134
  defined, 134
  example of, 136, 141, 142
  incongruence as sign of, 141
Psychotic groups, 76
Put-downs, 103

**R**

Rage, 49, 108, 132, 142
Reality testing, 16–17
Redecision therapy, 189, 197
Reframing of questions, 50–51
Regression in co-therapy, 80, 136–138, 143–144, 176
Reparenting, 133, 138–140, 149, 150–151
  boundaries, making of, 139
  defined, 133
  diagnosis, change of, 137
  dreams, 139
  mother, conflicting images of, 139
  new messages for patient, 138
  regression, 138
  therapeutic alliance, forming of, 139–140
Rescuer/Victim roles, 111–112
Resistance, working through in co-therapy, 6, 18, 27, 34, 77, 80, 117, 132, 137, 147, 150
Risk-taking in therapy, 18, 45, 61, 129
Rivalry between co-therapists, 102–103
Role models and modeling, 198–199, 207; *see also* Models and modeling
Rosenbaum, Max, 28, 30

**S**

Satir, Virginia, 2, 6, 69, 86, 120, 210–221; *see also* Therapists as models
Scapegoating, 43–44, 108, 146
  of assistant therapist, 43–44
  choice of one therapist as "trustworthy" one, 110–111
  of co-therapist, 109–110
Schilder, Paul, 6
Schizophrenia, 46–47, 108

theories about, 218
treatment of child in family, 46–47
Seduction, 47–48, 119, 122
by assistant therapist, 47–48
by co-therapist, 119
by patient, 122
Self; *see also* Boundaries
boundaries of, 206
representation, 131
revealing of to co-therapist, 85
Self-disclosure
as desirable quality in therapist, 64
modeling of, 34
Self-esteem, 13, 66
of co-therapist, 13, 173, 175, 212
Self-worth, 221
Sensitivity, 65, 67
Session spillover, 123–124
Sex of co-therapist as choice criterion,
68–69
Sex therapists, 34, 124; *see also*
Co-therapists
Sex-linked behavior, modeling of, 69
Sexual dysfunction, benefits of
opposite-sex teams for, 34
Sexual relationship of co-therapists,
open; *see also* Co-therapists
in group therapy, 33
married couples as model, 33, 34
sexual dysfunction, dealing with,
33, 34
and transference, 32–33
Sexual relationship of co-therapists,
secret, 31–32, 125–128; *see also*
Co-therapists
acting out conflicts, 125–126
co-dependency, 128
dismissal, risk of, 126–127
duties, distraction from, 127
example, 126
undermining of co-therapy by, 126
Sexuality, coping with issues in group
therapy, 33
Sharing of interventions and treatment
decisions, 25
Shaskan, Donald, 6
Splitting, 133, 134–135, 138, 143,
148, 151, 166, 167
awareness of, 134–135
of co-therapy team by patient, 134
defined, 134
Staff, problems of, 178
Stealing of patient, 231

Strokes and stroking, 81–82, 86, 132,
148, 194
and communication, 81–82
of co-therapists in session, 81–82
defined, 81
modeling of, 194
mutual, 86
Substance abuse, co-therapy group
for, 99
Suicide, attempted, 53, 93
Supervisors
boundaries of, 54
of co-learners, rules for, 41, 42–43,
171–172
commitment of, 62, 67
competition with, 57–58
contract for co-learners, sample,
234–235
of co-therapists, rules for, 98,
171–172
and countertransference, 59–60
of nequipos, rules for, 41–43,
171–172
Supervisory session, length of after
treatment, 46
Support staff, training of members,
52–53


T


Taking away from other co-therapist,
avoidance of, 196
Talk, amount of, vs. silence, 104
Taping for self-assessment and feedback, 196, 202
Task leadership role, 163
Team, *see* Co-therapists, relationship
issues; Co-therapist group issues
Termination, 15–16, 45, 73, 107, 117
of co-learner contract, 45
of co-therapy contract by
co-therapists, 73
lack of co-therapists' congruence
about, 117
loss, feelings of, arising from, premature, 15–16
Therapeutic alliance, 139–140, 148
Therapists as models, Satir's views on;
*see also* Models and modeling
clarity, 213
congruence, 211
husband/wife teams, 215

knowledge, actual, of therapist, 211
male–female model, power in, 212
permission to man to be parent, 214
realism about self in co-therapists, 215
roles, 212
self-esteem, building of, 211, 213
value of person, 212
Therapists, qualities desired for co-therapy
compatible, equal in power, non-competitive, 64
equal in communicating and open-ness, 63
sensitivity, empathy, 65
similar theoretical orientation, 64
skills, 64
Third party consultation, 106
Timing and pacing of therapy, 27
Touch
modeling of, 34
rules about, 78
Trainee as apprentice, 212
Training and trainees for psychother-apy; see also Co-learners; Nequipos
distinguished from co-therapists, 38
learning contract, time term of, 39
research with trainees, 40–41
Transactional Analysis, 189, 191–192
Transference, 13–15, 32–33, 44, 56, 69, 77–78, 112, 122, 136, 139, 141–142, 148, 168, 196, 202–203, 209, 219; see also Countertransference
asking for by use of word "me," 202
and bonding of clients, 13–15
as delay to cure, in Gouldings' work, 203
dual, 133, 136
erotic, 122

implications for supervisor and student, 44, 58
in group, 56
negative, 90, 135–136, 203
Triad, primary, family as, 219–220
and parents, 219, 220
Satir, work of on, 219, 220
Trust, in co-therapy team, 180, 182

U

Unequal married teams, 35–36
Unethical behavior, 102
Unilateral decision making, 103–104
Unresolved family disputes of co-therapists, 107
Unresolved problems of co-therapists, 17

V

Value, notion of, 212
Variety of means and perspectives in co-therapy, 13, 23

W

Weakland, John, 218
Whitaker, Carl, 3, 18–19, 21–22
Withdrawal, 131, 133
Women, 19, 52, 53, 54, 66, 69, 120–122, 123, 151, 190, 198–199, 212
as clients, 120–121
disparaging message to, 105
co-leading with, 198–199
in family therapy, 120–121
groups for, 52, 54, 55–56, 197–199
and male superiority, notion of, 120
modeling for, 66, 198, 199
recognition of need for male model-ing, 69
self-acceptance of, 19